The Psych
of Pandem

The Psychology of Pandemics:

Preparing for the Next Global Outbreak of Infectious Disease

By

Steven Taylor

Cambridge
Scholars
Publishing

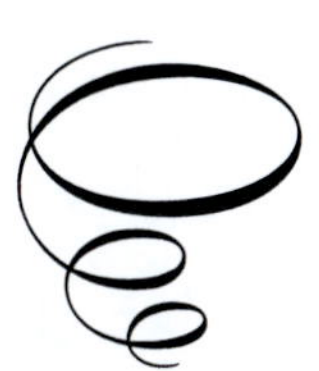

The Psychology of Pandemics:
Preparing for the Next Global Outbreak of Infectious Disease

By Steven Taylor

This book first published 2019. The present binding first published 2020.

Cambridge Scholars Publishing

Lady Stephenson Library, Newcastle upon Tyne, NE6 2PA, UK

British Library Cataloguing in Publication Data
A catalogue record for this book is available from the British Library

ISBN (10): 1-5275-4900-3
ISBN (13): 978-1-5275-4900-5

For Anna, Alex, and Meeru

Contents

FOREWORD

I've admired Dr. Taylor's work since I began reading it as a graduate student in the mid-1990s. His books and research articles on anxiety disorders stood out as particularly brilliant and eloquent. Inevitably, our paths began to cross as we attended the same professional conferences each year and were members of the Obsessive-Compulsive Cognitions Working Group (OCCWG) that formed in the late 1990s. But it was at one particular OCCWG meeting in 2001 in Whistler, British Columbia—and the ensuing World Congress of Cognitive Behavioral Therapy in Vancouver—where we developed the collaborative relationship that has remained to this day. And what a productive relationship it's been! As of this writing, we have published four books, 25 journal articles, and 22 book chapters together (most of them with a third colleague, Dr. Dean McKay). I have collaborated with countless colleagues on many research and writing projects, but Dr. Taylor tops them all when it comes to his astonishing mix of proficiency and efficiency.

So, what's a *psychologist* like Dr. Taylor doing writing a book about pandemics—a seemingly medical conundrum for biologists and physicians to sort out? I'll tell you what: He's synthesizing his interest in history, extensive grasp of research on social psychology and human behavior, and his substantial expertise on anxiety disorders to help us appreciate pandemics as a psychological problem as much as a medical one.

Communicable diseases existed during humankind's hunter-gatherer days. But it wasn't until about 10,000 years ago when we began living in communities and domesticating animals, that outbreaks of sicknesses such as malaria, tuberculosis, leprosy, influenza, smallpox, and others first appeared. Humans were blindsided, having little or no immunity to these viruses, and certainly no knowledge of how they could spread so easily (no one would propose that microorganisms caused these diseases until after 1000 AD). The more interactive human civilizations became—forming cities and establishing trade routes to connect with other cities—the more the probability of pandemics increased.

Fast forward to modernity, where people are exceedingly mobile and more likely to live in densely populated cities—factors that increase the risk of viruses spreading. Where hasty communication through a dizzying array of media also escalates the risk of panic and the chance that people who may be infected will travel in an attempt to avoid illness—potentially contributing to the spread of the virus. Months or years would go by before vaccines become available. In the meantime, clinics and hospitals would be overburdened, and there could be a lack of human resources to provide crucial services, due to both the demand and illness.

My point is that our behavior increases the chances of a pandemic… and our chances that if one occurred, it could be catastrophic.

And then there's the health anxiety factor—which Dr. Taylor knows so well from his decades of research on the topic. Such psychological elements often receive short-shrift when considered within the context of medical diseases. But the information age in which we currently live exposes us to so much data (and *distortions*) about health and illness it's not surprising we're vulnerable to overestimating our risk of, and vulnerability to, disease. Many of us try to cope with inaccurate beliefs about health and disease in ways that only strengthen such fears and lead them to persist and even spread. In turn, this leads to the kinds of unhealthy practices that may ironically aid the spread of the next pandemic.

Other clinical and social psychological factors that Dr. Taylor shows us are relevant for understanding pandemics include prejudices, the way we name diseases, the role of the media (not surprisingly, including social media), attitudes toward vaccinations, how we manage rumors, and the psychology of conspiracies. Synthesizing all of this, Dr. Taylor gives us a picture of how human factors impact the spreading of disease and emotional disturbance. He convinces us that knowledge of cognition and behavior will be critical for managing it—or, more optimistically, *preventing* it. Further, he proposes changes to public health policies and for how we can best exchange information about health risks.

In classic Steven Taylor style, this work is comprehensive, fusing viewpoints from multiple diverse disciplines. It is thoughtful and persuasive, grounded in scientific facts. And it has clear societal implications for us to heed. It also provides a call (and outline) for future research in medicine and clinical, health, and social psychology. As such, this book more than accomplishes its goals—it makes an exceptional contribution and fills a crucial gap in the literature on pandemics.

Jonathan S. Abramowitz, PhD
Professor of Psychology and Neuroscience
University of North Carolina at Chapel Hill

PREFACE

There have been numerous pandemics over the past century and earlier, typically arising from some form of influenza. Pandemic influenza is widely considered to be one of the leading public health threats facing the world today. Virologists predict that the next influenza pandemic could arrive any time in the coming years, with potentially devastating consequences. People do not have pre-existing immunity to the pathogens causing pandemics. Effective drug treatments are not always available. Vaccinations, if available, and behavioral methods are first-line interventions for reducing morbidity and mortality. Behavioral methods include hygienic practices (e.g., hand-washing) and social distancing methods (e.g., limiting large social gatherings).

The question arises as to how best apportion healthcare resources for managing pandemics. Such resources, by definition, are limited. It is important that resources be apportioned to essential services and to the development and distribution of vaccines and other methods for halting or limiting the spread of infection. Remarkably, public health agencies have devoted few resources for specifically dealing with the psychological factors that influence pandemic-related emotional reactions (e.g., fear, anxiety, distress) and behavioral problems (e.g., nonadherence, avoidance, stigmatization of out-groups). Healthcare authorities neglect the role of psychological factors in pandemic-related infection even though these factors are important for many reasons. They play a vital role, for example, in adherence to vaccination and social distancing, both of which are vital for stemming the spread of infection. Nonadherence to vaccination is a widespread problem even during pandemics.

Psychological factors also play an important role in the way in which people cope with the threat of pandemic infection and its sequelae, such as the loss of loved ones. Although many people cope well under threat, many other people experience high levels of distress or a worsening of pre-existing psychological problems, such as anxiety disorders and other clinical conditions. Psychological factors are further important for understanding and managing broader societal problems associated with pandemics, such as factors involved in the spreading of excessive fear. People may fear for their health, safety, family, finances, or jobs. Psychological factors are also important for understanding and managing the potentially disruptive or maladaptive defensive reactions, such as increases in stigmatization and xenophobia that occur when people are threatened with infection.

The purpose of this volume is to fill an important gap in the literature on pandemics. Goals are to (1) describe the psychological reactions to pandemics, including maladaptive behaviors and emotional and defensive reactions, (2) review the psychological vulnerability factors that contribute to the spreading of disease and emotional distress, (3) discuss empirically supported methods for addressing these psychological problems, and (4) outline the implications for public health policy, including implications for risk communication. Influenza pandemics are used as prototypic examples because they have been the most common pandemics over the past century and influenza is likely to be a source of future pandemics. Other disease outbreaks are discussed where relevant.

To achieve the aims of this volume, the author draws on sources from multiple disciplines, including virology, epidemiology, public health, sociology, history of medicine and, of course, psychology. Numerous subdisciplines within psychology are drawn upon, including clinical psychology, health psychology, and social psychology. In addition to drawing extensively from the research literature, case examples are included throughout this volume to highlight important issues.

About the Author

Steven Taylor, Ph.D., is a Professor and Clinical Psychologist in the Department of Psychiatry at the University of British Columbia, Vancouver, Canada. He received his B.Sc. (Hons.) and M.Sc. at the University of Melbourne, and Ph.D. at the University of British Columbia. Dr. Taylor's research and clinical work focuses largely on anxiety disorders and related clinical conditions, including fears and phobias, health anxiety, posttraumatic stress disorder, and obsessive-compulsive disorder. He has authored over 300 scientific publications and more than 20 books, which have been translated into several languages. His books include *Understanding and treating panic disorder* (John Wiley & Sons), *Treating health anxiety* (Guilford Publications), and *Clinician's Guide to Posttraumatic Stress Disorder* (Guilford Publications). Dr. Taylor was a member of the anxiety disorders committee for the text revision of the fourth edition of the *Diagnostic and Statistical Manual of Mental Disorders*. He has also served as Editor or Associate Editor of several academic journals, including *Behaviour Research and Therapy, Journal of Cognitive Psychotherapy*, and the *Journal of Obsessive-Compulsive and Related Disorders*. Dr. Taylor has received a number of awards for his scholarly work, including awards from the Canadian Psychological Association, Association for Advancement of Behavior Therapy, and the Anxiety Disorders Association of America. In addition to teaching and research, Dr. Taylor maintains a clinical practice in Vancouver, BC, specializing in mood and anxiety disorders.

Acronyms used throughout this volume

BIS	Behavioral immune system
CBT	Cognitive-behavior therapy
CDC	Centers for Disease Control and Prevention
HCW	Healthcare worker
HIV	Human immunodeficiency virus
PTSD	Posttraumatic stress disorder
PVD	Perceived vulnerability to disease
PVDS	Perceived Vulnerability to Disease Scale
SARS	Severe acute respiratory syndrome
WHO	World Health Organization

CHAPTER 1

WHAT IS A PANDEMIC?

Overview

> Despite the passage of decades, 96-year-old James S. vividly recalled the 1918 Spanish flu pandemic. He was 8 years old at the time. The city had ground to a halt. Schools and theaters were closed, and dances and other social gatherings were banned. James was not even allowed to go to the local playground because his father feared he would fall ill. Church services were banned, despite protests from the clergy. James recalled the pine caskets in the front room of the family home, containing the bodies of his mother and younger sister. It all happened so quickly; people could fall sick in the morning and be dead by evening. People were afraid to leave their homes, he recalled, although it was necessary for the government to impose fines if an infected person was out in public, because some sick people refused to stay indoors.

Pandemic influenza is one of the leading health threats currently facing the world (World Health Organization (WHO), 2019). The rise of antimicrobial resistance, along with the emergence of new, highly pathogenic viral strains, has fueled fears of another global outbreak of infectious disease (Nerlich & Halliday, 2007). For pandemics in general, the causal elements are manifold and complex. The essential elements are an infectious agent (e.g., a virus or bacterium), a host (e.g., a person), and the environment. The host's resistance to infection depends on several factors including immunocompetence as well as psychological factors that influence how the host copes with or reacts to threatened or actual infection. Environmental factors are numerous and multiform, including factors that promote or hamper the coping strategies of the host.

This book focuses on the psychological factors as they pertain to the host and host-environment interactions in pandemics. Put simply, pandemics of infectious disease are not just events in which some infectious "bug" spreads throughout the world. Pandemics are events in which the population's psychological reactions to infection play an essential role in both the spreading and containment of the disease, and influence the extent to which widespread emotional distress and social disorder occur. When threatened with infection, people vary widely in their reactions. The complexities of their reactions need to be taken into consideration in order to understand the psychology of pandemics. The present volume aims to explore these issues through a review of the scientific and historical literatures, supplemented by illustrative case vignettes derived from various sources including historical sources and the author's clinical case files. This book also considers the public health implications for assessing and addressing pandemic-related emotional distress, and for addressing pandemic-related social or behavioral problems, such as vaccination nonadherence.

The focus of this book is on influenza pandemics because influenza is the most likely source of the next pandemic. However, findings from other pertinent outbreaks, such as Severe Acute Respiratory Syndrome (SARS), Bubonic Plague, Ebola virus disease, and others, are discussed where relevant.

Definition

Pandemics are large-scale epidemics afflicting millions of people across multiple countries, sometimes spreading throughout the globe (WHO, 2010b). For a virus or bacterium to cause a pandemic it must be an organism for which most people do not have preexisting immunity, transmitting easily from person to person, and causing severe illness (Kilbourne, 1977). Diseases causing pandemics are part of a group of conditions known as emerging infectious diseases (Lederberg, Shope, & Oakes, 1992), which include newly identified pathogens as well as reemerging ones.

Notable Pandemics

The most famous pandemic was the Bubonic Plague (e.g., 1346-1353), attributed to *Yersinia pestis*, which killed an estimated 50 million people worldwide (Johnson & Mueller, 2002). Over the past century, there have been many other pandemics of varying degrees of contagiousness and lethality. Examples include HIV/AIDS (1981 to present), the Spanish flu (a strain of the H1N1 influenza virus; 1918-1920), Russian flu (H2N2 or H3N8, 1889-1890), Asian flu (H2N2, 1957-1958), Hong Kong flu (H3N2, 1968-1969), a second Russian flu pandemic (H1N1, 1977-1978), Swine flu (H1N1, 2009-2010), and the Zika virus pandemic (2015-2016) (Belshe, 2005; Crosby, 2003; Doherty, 2013; Honigsbaum, 2014; Morens & Fauci, 2017; WHO, 2010b). Avian flu has been widespread in recent years but at the time of writing has not reached pandemic proportions.

Nomenclature

The notation system for influenza, H*x*N*x* (e.g., H1N1, H3N8) refers to the virus's hemagglutinin (H) and neuraminidase (N) membrane proteins. Terms such as "Swine flu" and "Asian flu" have become standard labels for pandemics. Such names are used here because readers will likely be familiar with them. However, as we will see later, such terms should be used with caution. The terms "flu" and "influenza" also can be sources of confusion. With the exception of the established names for pandemics (e.g., "Swine flu"), the term "influenza" rather than "flu" will be used throughout this book because "flu" is a vague, broad term used to describe symptoms and signs that may or may not be caused by an influenza virus (e.g., fever, cough, runny nose, muscle aches; Doshi, 2013).

Pandemic Influenza

Pandemics are usually viral in nature, typically arising from animal influenza viruses that spread to humans (WHO, 2010b). It is difficult to predict when the next influenza pandemic will occur.

> Despite continuing progress in many areas, including enhanced human and animal surveillance and large-scale viral genomic screening, we are probably no better able today to anticipate and prevent the emergence of pandemic influenza than 5 centuries ago, as shown by the completely unexpected emergence of the 2009 novel H1N1 pandemic virus. (Morens, Taubenberger, Folkers, & Fauci, 2010, p. 1444)

It has been speculated that future pandemics will arise from some strain of Avian influenza (e.g., H5N1 or H7N9) or from combinations of

Avian and other influenza strains (Kelland, 2017; Li et al., 2010; Webster & Govorkova, 2006; Wildoner, 2016). The next influenza pandemic is inevitable and serious (Laver & Webster, 2001; Webby & Webster, 2003).

> The world's population would have no immunity to this "new" virus. Because of today's crowded conditions and with modern rapid transportation facilities, the epidemic would spread like wildfire, reaching every corner of the globe. Many millions of people would become ill and there would certainly be many deaths. (Laver & Webster, 2001, p. 1813)

The frequent genetic mutation and genetic reassortment of influenza viruses make it difficult, if not impossible, to prevent influenza pandemics from occurring (Kelland, 2017). Compounding the problem, viral pandemics, just like comparatively smaller-scale epidemics, are often followed by secondary bacterial infection (e.g., hospital-acquired pneumonia), thereby complicating treatment and increasing the risk of mortality (Morens et al., 2010). Indeed, 95% of post-mortem samples from the Spanish flu pandemic showed bacterial infection complications, and the majority of deaths likely resulted from secondary bacterial pneumonia caused by common upper respiratory tract bacteria (Morens, Taubenberger, & Fauci, 2008).

Influenza pandemics and seasonal influenza have some similarities but important differences. Pandemic influenza can arise during the usual influenza season—that is, the winter months in temperate climates—but can also occur during the summer (Taubenberger & Morens, 2006). Pandemic influenza, by definition, spreads globally (i.e., is more transmissible; Fraser et al., 2009), is often (but not always) more lethal (Doherty, 2013), and can differ from seasonal influenza in terms of the people most severely afflicted. Seasonal influenza tends to be most dangerous to the elderly and medically frail, whereas some influenza pandemics have taken the greatest toll on other age groups. To illustrate, consider the Spanish flu, which killed 20% of those infected (Taubenberger & Morens, 2006), with an estimated death toll of 35-100 million people worldwide, or 2-6% of the world's population (Barry, 2009; Johnson & Mueller, 2002). The Spanish flu was most lethal to children and young adults (Taubenberger & Morens, 2006). Similarly, young adults were more susceptible to Swine flu than older adults (Crum-Cianflone et al., 2009).

Some pandemics killed with great rapidity. In the case of the Spanish flu, there were numerous accounts of people waking up sick in the morning and dying later that day, on their way to work, for example (Crosby, 2003; Pettigrew, 1983). The deaths were sometimes gruesome. Some victims of the Spanish flu developed pulmonary edema and became so anoxic that their faces turned blue. Some of these patients hemorrhaged from the mucous membranes, particularly the nose, stomach, and intestines, and there was also bleeding from the ears and petechial (skin) hemorrhages (Taubenberger, Reid, Janczewski, & Fanning, 2001).

Pandemic-Related Stressors

Pandemics are "frequently marked by uncertainty, confusion and a sense of urgency" (WHO, 2005, p. 1). Prior to, or in the early stages of a pandemic, there is widespread uncertainty about the odds and seriousness of becoming infected, along with uncertainty, and possible misinformation, about the best methods of prevention and management (Kanadiya & Sallar, 2011). Uncertainty may persist well into the pandemic, especially concerning the question of whether a pandemic is truly over. Pandemics can come in waves (Barry, 2005; Caley, Philp, & McCracken, 2008; Herrera-Valdez, Cruz-Aponte, & Castillo-Chavez, 2011). Waves of infection are caused, in part, by fluctuations in patterns of human aggregation, such as seasonal movements of people away from, and then into contact with, one another (e.g., schools closing for the summer and then reopening), as well as other fluctuations in social aggregation (Caley et al., 2008; Herrera-Valdez et al., 2011). The Spanish flu, for example, came in three waves (Barry, 2005). Accordingly, there may be uncertainty as to whether a pandemic has truly run its course.

Pandemics are associated with a score of other psychosocial stressors, including health threats to oneself and loved ones. There may be severe disruptions of routines, separation from family and friends, shortages of food and medicine, wage loss, social isolation due to quarantine or other social distancing programs, and school closure (Shultz, Espinel, Flynn, Hoffmann, & Cohen, 2008). Families may become malnourished if no one in the house is well enough to shop or cook (Schoch-Spana, 2004). Personal financial hardship can occur if a family's primary wage earner is unable to work because of illness. During the Spanish flu, for example, merchants suffered hardship because of staff absenteeism and because shoppers were either too ill or too frightened to venture out to the stores (Pettigrew, 1983). The personal financial impact of a pandemic can be as severe and stressful as the infection itself, especially for people who are already experiencing financial hardship. This is illustrated by the following account of one American family during the Spanish flu pandemic.

> In December 1918 influenza struck, infecting Mr. D. and then his wife and five children. By late December he had been out of work for three weeks due to his own illness and then that of his family. For the first few weeks the family had managed on their meager savings and on money sent from a relative. After that, the family became frantic and approached the *Society of the Friendless* for aid. Mr. D. was unable to go to work because he dared not leave his sick family unattended. The situation became increasingly desperate. They had run out of coal for heating and there was no food in the house. Having no money, Mr. D. attempted to get credit at the grocery store but was declined. Compounding his problems, Mr. D. lost his job because of his absence from work. (Bristow, 2010, pp. 139-140)

During a pandemic, people may be exposed to the death of friends and loved ones, including exposure to the death of children. The latter can be especially traumatizing (Taylor, 2017). Caring for the sick can be highly stressful, especially if this burden falls on children, as illustrated by the following example from Britain, during the Spanish flu.

> Writing from Coventry in 1973, Ethel Robson recalled how at the age of nine she was suddenly thrust into the role of sole caretaker for her family when her eight brothers and sisters, ranging in ages from 10 months to 15 years, contracted the flu together with her mother. For some reason, Robson writes, "I was the only one out of all the family that didn't have the virus." Although a doctor visited twice a day, no one else was allowed into the house, "therefore I was doing my best to help the others." (Honigsbaum, 2009, p. 86)

Most of Robson's siblings recovered but her seven-year-old sister and mother died. "It really was a terrible time not knowing who we were going to lose next," she recalled (Honigsbaum, 2009, p. 86).

The following account from northern Labrador (Canada), during the Spanish flu pandemic, was provided by the Reverend Walter Perrett, concerning an eight-year-old girl, whose parents and siblings had died from influenza, leaving the young girl alone to fend for herself for five weeks before being found.

> The huskies (dogs) now began to eat the dead bodies, and the child was a spectator of this horrible incident. So mad did the beasts become, upon taking human flesh, that they attacked the child herself, biting her arm. ... It was thirty degrees below zero. The little girl had used the last of the Christmas candles to melt snow for drinking water (Pettigrew, 1983, pp. 29-30).

A pandemic can impede a community's ability to bury the dead according to accepted cultural and religious practices. During the Spanish flu pandemic, there were shortages of coffins and insufficient funeral staff to prepare and bury bodies (Johnson, 2006). Handling of the deceased is an emotionally charged issue, and neglect of customary, culturally prescribed, funerary practices can be experienced as abhorrent and dehumanizing (Schoch-Spana, 2004).

Indirect exposure to trauma, such as graphic media depictions of fatalities, can also contribute to distress (Neria & Sullivan, 2011). Other stressors include the loss or destruction of possessions. When people are forced to evacuate their homes, leaving their possessions behind, looting can occur (Staino, 2008).

Cultural minorities residing within a larger mainstream culture, such as new immigrants, may experience stressors that are not encountered by people from the majority culture, such as unfamiliarity with community support systems, difficulty accessing services due to language difficulties, discrimination, and immigration status issues. Thus, during times of pandemic, some ethnic minorities may experience more adverse psychological consequences than members from the majority culture (Shultz et al., 2008).

Effects on the Healthcare System

Pandemics can exceed the capacities of healthcare systems to care for the sick. This is for various reasons including widespread infection, lack of effective treatment, and breakdown of the healthcare system due to healthcare workers (HCWs) becoming infected and unable to care for the ill (National Academy of Medicine, 2016). Failure to manage the surge of people into hospitals and clinics can create unnecessary exposure to disease as infected and non-infected persons congregate to seek services and treatments (Shultz et al., 2008). Sick people may be turned away from overcrowded, short-staffed hospitals, thereby necessitating home care (Schoch-Spana, 2004). This can create a financial burden in arranging home care for a sick family member.

Economic Costs

Pandemics can have major effects on the broader economy and societal infrastructure. As people become ill and unable to fulfill their occupational roles, essential services may break down (Shultz, Baingana, & Neria, 2015). In Baltimore during the Spanish flu, for example, garbage piled up in the streets due to absenteeism of sanitation personnel (Schoch-Spana, 2004). This created further public health problems. Even with effective vaccines and antiviral medications, it has been estimated that the next influenza pandemic could result in economic losses of over US$34 billion in the United States (Prager, Wei, & Rose, 2017). Worldwide, it has been estimated that the next pandemic could cost over US$6 trillion in economic losses (National Academy of Medicine, 2016).

How do Pandemics Spread?

Human networks are the major means of pandemic disease transmission (Wald, 2008). Influenza is readily spread by inhaling airborne cough or sneeze droplets, and by touching one's mouth, nose, or eyes after touching fomites. The latter are contaminated surfaces in public spaces, such as doors, railings, or tabletops, or contaminated objects such as toys, doorknobs, and banknotes (Nicas & Jones, 2009; Thomas et al., 2008). Airborne transmission, combined with high population densities in urban areas and the availability of modern rapid transportation, makes it easy for influenza infection to spread rapidly.

Some people disproportionately contribute to the spreading of infection. These people are known as superspreaders (Galvani & May, 2005). In prototypic cases of superspreading as few as 20% of infected people may be responsible for 80% of transmissions (Woolhouse et al., 1997). A superspreader is likely to be someone who (1) is not immunized or is immunocompromised and therefore particularly susceptible to infection, (2) does not engage in basic hygiene (e.g., covering coughs) and therefore likely to transmit influenza, (3) comes into contact with a great many people, through some combination of their social and occupational roles (e.g., a flight attendant, cafeteria worker, or someone with a highly active social life), or comes into regular contact with sick people that are particularly susceptible to infection (e.g., a hospital worker that deals with patients but refuses to be vaccinated) (Galvani & May, 2005; Shen et al., 2004; Temime et al., 2009).

Superspreading is also shaped by other factors, including the nature of the infectious agent and herd immunity. Herd immunity, also known as community immunity, refers to the indirect protection from infectious disease that occurs when a large proportion of the population becomes immune to infection, which provides a degree of protection to people who are not immune (Fine, Eames, & Heymann, 2011). This impedes the spread of infection by disrupting the chains of contagion.

Superspreading is especially likely to occur for diseases that have substantial incubation periods; that is, periods in which infected people are contagious but asymptomatic, meaning that the person may be unknowingly spreading disease to others. Incubation periods for influenza may vary from person to person (Virlogeux et al., 2016) and may depend on the strain. During the 2009 Swine flu pandemic, the incubation period was 1-4 days (Nishiura & Inaba, 2011; Tuite et al., 2010). A study conducted in China during the Avian flu epidemic found that the median incubation period was 8 days (Huang et al., 2014). Such a long incubation period means that a person may infect many other people before becoming symptomatic.

The 2003 SARS outbreak is an example in which superspreading was well-documented (Shen et al., 2004). SARS, which spreads in a manner similar to influenza, can have an incubation period of 2-10 days (Shen et al., 2004). In one case of SARS superspreading, a 62-year-old woman was admitted to a Beijing hospital for treatment of diabetes mellitus. While in hospital, her SARS symptoms became apparent (e.g., fever, headache) but were misdiagnosed as tuberculosis. Her clinical condition deteriorated and she died. During her hospital stay, she had 74 close contacts, including 25 HCWs, 11 relatives, 36 co-patients in the same ward, and 2 people who accompanied other patients on the ward. Among these close contacts, SARS developed in 33 (45%) of the 74 people (Shen et al., 2004). Superspreaders have also been reported for many other outbreaks of infectious disease, such as the Middle East Respiratory Syndrome Coronavirus (e.g., Al-Tawfiq & Memish, 2016; Lau et al., 2017).

Historically, the most famous superspreader was Mary Mallon, dubbed "Typhoid Mary" by the news media (Soper, 1939). Typhoid is a highly contagious infectious disease caused by *Salmonella typhi*. People can be chronically asymptomatic carriers (Wain, Hendriksen, Mikoleit, Keddy, & Ochiai, 2015). At the turn of the 20th century, typhoid epidemics were commonplace, with no effective treatment (Soper,

1939). From 1902-1909, Mallon, a chronic but asymptomatic carrier, infected more than 50 people with typhoid before she was involuntarily quarantined in a hospital for communicable diseases in New York. What made her case tragic was that she stubbornly refused to give up working as a cook, despite being infected, which led to her involuntary confinement. It was quite obvious that Mallon was infecting people. Each time she moved to a new house to serve as a household cook, the occupants became sick. Never staying long, she moved from house to house, gaining her employment through job placement agencies. Mallon adamantly denied being infected, even after infecting so many people and being involuntarily quarantined.

> The authorities offered to release Mallon [from quarantine] if she would agree to give up professional cooking or have her gall bladder removed, since it was believed [erroneously] to be the site of her chronic infection. She rejected both offers, and denied that she was responsible for anyone's sickness or death. She refused to recognize the authority of science or government to label her a menace to society. ... "I never had typhoid in my life, and have always been healthy," Mallon told one reporter. "Why should I be banished like a leper and compelled to live in solitary confinement with only a dog for a companion?" (Brooks, 1996, p. 916)

Mallon was released on the proviso that she promised not to work as a cook, not to handle the food of others, observe various other precautions, and report to the New York City Department of Health every three months (Soper, 1939). But on release, she promptly disappeared, changed her name, and resumed working as a cook in hotels, restaurants, and sanatoria. While working at a maternity hospital she infected 25 people. She was later apprehended and returned to the quarantine hospital, where she spent the remainder of her life (Brooks, 1996).

The case of Typhoid Mary is relevant to a future influenza pandemic in that it is possible that some people will be asymptomatic carriers of influenza. As many as 36% of people infected with seasonal influenza may be asymptomatic and never show symptoms, possibly due to preexisting partial immunity (Furuya-Kanamori et al., 2016). Such people can inadvertently transmit the virus to other people, but not at the same rate as symptomatic people (Bridges, Kuehnert, & Hall, 2003).

Mary Mallon adamantly denied that she was inflected with typhoid, and so her spreading of typhoid did not appear to be intentional. But what about the intentional spread of infection? There have been numerous cases of people deliberately spreading infection during pandemics, such as HIV-positive people deliberately or recklessly infecting others (e.g., BBC News, 2001; Hammond, Holmes, & Mercier, 2016; Wainberg, 2008; Watt, 2017). Several writers have speculated that influenza could be deliberately spread as part of a bioterrorist attack (e.g., Krug, 2003; Lutz, Bronze, & Greenfield, 2003; Quick, 2018; Ricks, 2003; Wiwanitkit, 2015). To date, however, there have been no documented accounts of people deliberately spreading influenza. Unintentional spreading of infection due to poor hygiene (e.g., neglecting to cover coughs) and lack of vaccination is a more likely way in which influenza will be disseminated during the next pandemic.

Socioeconomic Factors

How do socioeconomic factors influence the odds of infection and distress? Although some accounts of the Spanish flu claimed that the poor succumbed as readily as the rich (Crosby, 2003), later research suggests that the first wave of infection primarily affected the poor, whereas people from the upper social classes were more afflicted by the second wave (Mamelund, 2018). Something similar happened during the Bubonic Plague in the 16th century. Wealthy citizens fled the infected cities to their countryside villas (Cohn, 2010). This had two effects. First, the poorer people who were left behind were disproportionately more likely to be infected, at least initially, since they remained in the infected cities. Second, the wealthy, by fleeing from the cities, brought plague to the countryside.

> The poor may have been among the first victims but the pestilence eventually levelled populations equally ... Few saw the rich surviving any better than the poor. (Cohn, 2010, p. 208)

There are several possible reasons why the poor were among the first victims, including overcrowding, which increases the risk of contagion, poor housing conditions, lack of access to clean water (increasing the risk of secondary infection), and being in poor health before they were struck by infection (O'Sullivan & Phillips, 2019). People with greater economic resources have great opportunities for seeking medical care and for avoiding infection, at least in the short term, including fleeing infected areas until the pandemic catches up with them. The same thing may happen during the next pandemic. Depopulation of cities occurred in past pandemics and could occur during the next one. The historical record, although scant in details, suggests that both wealthy and poor people will be at risk for pandemic-related psychological distress.

Goals of this Volume

As is evident from this introductory chapter, this book contains numerous case reports and historical descriptions. These are not simply "stories"; they are important examples of how people have reacted to pandemics and other outbreaks. People are often myopic in their threat appraisals; focusing on immediate concerns, rapidly forgetting the lessons of the past, and neglecting to anticipate long-term potential dangers. Indeed, it has been observed that many people too quickly forget things like epidemics or pandemics (Crosby, 2003; Quick, 2018). Case examples and historical depictions help to vividly portray what it is like to live during times of pandemic. Armed with such knowledge, we are better able to anticipate and prepare for the next pandemic.

Contemporary guidelines and approaches to managing pandemics have focused primarily on limiting the spread of infection. Health authorities have devoted relatively little attention to identifying and managing psychological factors likely to influence the spreading of emotional distress and infection (Douglas, Douglas, Harrigan, & Douglas, 2009; Shultz et al., 2008). This is revealed in the lack of attention to mental health issues in pandemic preparedness documents (e.g., Centers for Disease Control and Prevention (CDC), 2007; Pan-Canadian Public Health Network, 2016; WHO, 2005). This is a remarkable omission given that vaccination nonadherence and related issues are essentially psychological problems, driven by people's beliefs and expectations. Psychological factors are relevant to behavioral methods of disease containment (e.g., hygiene and social distancing) and for managing emotional distress and maladaptive or disruptive behaviors that can occur during times of pandemic. Accordingly, these are the points of focus in the present volume.

In the remaining chapters we will (1) review the nature and importance of psychological reactions during pandemics, including emotional reactions and maladaptive behaviors, (2) examine the theory and research relevant for understanding psychological reactions to pandemics, at both an individual and societal level, (3) discuss empirically supported methods for addressing these psychological factors, and (4) describe the implications for public health policy, including implications for risk communication and issues for further investigation. As mentioned, the focus is primarily on influenza pandemics, although other infectious disease outbreaks will be discussed as relevant.

CHAPTER 2

CONTEMPORARY METHODS FOR MANAGING PANDEMICS

Overview

Preparation for a pandemic involves considerable time and planning. Contemporary influenza plans (e.g., CDC, 2007; WHO, 2005) begin with disease forecasting and surveillance (e.g., influenza forecasting programs) to track the occurrence of outbreaks. This is followed by an assessment of the likely risks and probable need for resources, and plans for the optimal allocation of resources (e.g., vaccine prioritization to particular segments of the population). Four main methods are used to manage the spread of infection: (1) Risk communication (public education), (2) vaccines and antiviral therapies, (3) hygiene practices, and (4) social distancing (WHO, 2008, 2012; WHO Writing Group, 2006). Psychological factors play an essential role in the success of each of these methods.

Risk Communication

During a pandemic, the overriding public health goal is to bring the outbreak under control as quickly as possible with minimal disruption. Effective risk communication is essential for achieving this goal (Barry, 2009). Health authorities have been criticized for their lack of attention to risk communication.

> In the face of an epidemic, terror, blame, rumors, and conspiracy theories, distrust in authorities, and panic can take hold simultaneously. This is why establishing and maintaining trust through honest, clear communication is paramount. History continues to show us that health communication lies at the heart of epidemic control, yet staffing for such communication is usually tacked onto health budgets as an afterthought, at woefully inadequate levels. (Quick, 2018, p. 150).

Risk communication involves giving the public the information they need to make well-informed decisions about how to protect their health and safety. Important elements of the WHO (2005, 2008) communication guidelines are as follows:

1. Announce the outbreak early, even with incomplete information, so as to minimize the spread of rumors and misinformation.
2. Provide information about what the public can do to make themselves safer.
3. Maintain transparency to ensure public trust.
4. Demonstrate that efforts are being made to understand the public's views and concerns about the outbreak.
5. Evaluate the impact of communication programs to ensure that the messages are being correctly understood and that the advice is being followed.

Although the WHO guidelines might appear sound and might seem to address psychological issues in risk communication, there are important issues that are not addressed. For example, is adherence to health guidelines improved by messages that induce fear in the public, or do such messages tend to backfire? Such psychological issues merit careful consideration and are discussed later in this volume.

Pharmacological Treatments

Vaccines and antiviral medications are the primary pharmacological methods for managing pandemic influenza. The development of vaccines for infectious diseases is a time consuming, costly business, with a more than 90% failure rate (Gouglas et al., 2018). In other words, the overwhelming majority of experimental vaccines prove to be ineffective. During the Spanish flu pandemic, experimental vaccines were developed on the erroneous assumption that the Spanish flu was bacterial in nature (Pettigrew, 1983). The availability of a plethora of experimental vaccines during that pandemic created confusion for the public, medical practitioners, and health authorities (Heagerty, 1919). Today, even successful vaccines provide only partial protection against infection. But that is better than no protection at all.

Antiviral medications are used to treat influenza and to provide prophylaxis to exposed persons. Antivirals, particularly neuraminidase inhibitors such as oseltamivir (Tamiflu), may be effective against the next strain of pandemic influenza because of the track record of these drugs in previous influenza outbreaks (Beard, Brendish, & Clark, 2018). However, their efficacy in the next pandemic is by no means certain because of the possible emergence of resistant strains. To complicate matters, population-based simulation studies suggest that under certain conditions, neuraminidase prophylaxis could have paradoxical effects, promoting the occurrence and transmission of neuraminidase resistant strains of influenza (Eichner et al., 2009).

As noted in Chapter 1, evidence suggests that the majority of Spanish flu fatalities were due to secondary bacterial pneumonia. Therefore, antibiotics will likely play an important role in managing the next pandemic. An issue of concern is the rise of antibiotic-resistant bacteria. The growing prevalence of such bacteria could increase the toll of future pandemics, even if those pandemics are viral in origin (Megiddo et al., 2019).

Although there has been some debate as to the safety and efficacy of seasonal influenza vaccines (Alcalde-Cabero et al., 2016; Babcock, Jernigan, & Relman, 2014; Doshi, 2013, 2014), health authorities continue to emphasize the importance of vaccination for both seasonal and pandemic influenza (CDC, 2018b; WHO, 2012). Vaccines might not be suitable for all members of the population and there may be a risk of adverse effects, such as Guillain Barré Syndrome. However, such complications are rare. It has been estimated that only one or two new cases of Guillain Barré Syndrome occur in every million doses of influenza vaccine (CDC, 2018a). Some critics have argued that vaccination for measles, mumps, and rubella increases the risk of autism, but this has been debunked because the claim was based on flawed and fraudulent research (Godlee, Smith, & Marcovitch, 2011). Unfortunately, however, the link between this vaccine and autism, although bogus, garnered a good deal of media attention, thereby fueling fears about vaccines in general, including influenza vaccines.

A potential problem with influenza vaccines is that they might not be available in the early stage of the next pandemic. Even if effective vaccines are developed, there may be an insufficient supply due to demand exceeding production capacity (Oshitani, 2006). Willingness to be vaccinated is also a major issue affecting the success of vaccination programs. Most people do *not* adhere to vaccination recommendations. For example, only about 30% of US adults routinely receive vaccination against seasonal influenza (Levi, Segal, St. Laurent, & Lieberman, 2010). During the Swine flu pandemic in 2009, fewer than 40% of people in the US, UK, and Canada sought, or intended to seek, vaccination (CDC,

2011; Statistics Canada, 2010; SteelFisher et al., 2012; Taha, Matheson, & Anisman, 2013). In a study conducted in Switzerland during the same pandemic, no more than 20% of the population sought vaccination (Bangerter et al., 2012). Psychological factors, as discussed later in this book, are important for understanding seemingly self-defeating behaviors such as vaccination nonadherence.

Hygiene Practices

Commonly recommended hygiene practices include handwashing with soap or hand sanitizer, covering sneezes/coughs (e.g., sneezing into the crook of one's arm), hand awareness (i.e., refraining from touching one's eyes, nose or mouth), cleaning household surfaces, and wearing facemasks (Aiello et al., 2010; WHO, 2008). Research indicates that the spread of respiratory viruses can be reduced by frequent handwashing (Jefferson et al., 2011). There is insufficient evidence to determine whether efficacy is improved by using viricidals or antiseptics instead of plain soap (Jefferson et al., 2011).

Facemasks were widely used during the Spanish flu pandemic, and indeed the wearing of protective facemasks was mandated by law in many places (Arnold, 2018b). Today, the evidence for the efficacy of facemasks for the general public is mixed (Cowling et al., 2008), although N95 respirator facemasks might provide some degree of protection against airborne pathogens (WHO, 2008). Facemasks are more important in limiting the spread of infection in hospital settings (Jefferson et al., 2011).

Regarding acceptability, practices such as covering coughs, handwashing, and using soap are typically acceptable to the general public, whereas masks tend to be less acceptable, particularly in Western countries (Aiello et al., 2010; Stebbins, Downs, & Vukotich, 2009; SteelFisher et al., 2012). An unintended consequence of facemasks is that the sight of people wearing masks might heighten anxiety by serving as reminders of health-related threats (Wald, 2008).

Although handwashing is generally acceptable among people as a means of reducing the spread of disease, this does not necessarily translate into actual washing behaviors. Despite public health warnings, people routinely fail to adhere to handwashing recommendations, particularly if they are not being observed by others (Pfattheicher, Strauch, Diefenbacher, & Schnuerch, 2018). For example, it is common for people to fail to wash their hands after using the toilet. To illustrate, a British study found that a quarter of rail and bus commuters had fecal bacteria on their hands (Judah et al., 2010). According to a systematic review of 96 studies, a mean of 40% of people fail to wash their hands after toilet use (Erasmus et al., 2010). During the 2009 Swine flu pandemic, people who viewed themselves as having a low risk of infection were less likely to wash their hands (Gilles et al., 2011). As discussed later in this book, several psychological variables predict a person's proclivity to engage in the hygiene behaviors necessary for pandemic control.

Social Distancing

Social distancing refers to interventions, either recommended or mandated by health authorities, to reduce the probability that infected people will spread disease to others (Finkelstein, Prakash, Nigmatulina, Klaiman, & Larson, 2010). Social distancing can include some or all of the following, depending on the severity of an outbreak: Quarantine of infected persons, school closure, workplace closure, cancelling mass gatherings such as sporting events and concerts, closing recreational facilities (e.g., community centers), closing non-essential businesses (e.g., clubs and bars), cancelling non-essential domestic travel, self-imposed isolation of uninfected people (e.g., remaining home, when possible), and border and travel restrictions (Pan-Canadian Public Health Network, 2016; WHO, 2010b). Increasing interpersonal space has also been suggested; for example, keeping a distance of 1-2 meters from people who show signs of infection (Pan-Canadian Public Health Network, 2016; WHO, 2010a).

Social distancing must be applied immediately, rigorously, and consistently to be effective (Maharaj & Kleczkowski, 2012). Social distancing is especially important for children and teenagers (e.g., school closure and keeping children and teens at home), because these age groups disproportionately contribute to the spread of infection (Cauchemez et al., 2009; CDC, 2007; Fraser et al., 2009; Stebbins et al., 2009). According to the CDC (2007), "schools ... serve as amplification points of seasonal community influenza epidemics, and children are thought to play a significant role in introducing and transmitting the influenza virus" (p. 27). Thus, schools and preschools are "hot spots" for the dissemination of influenza (Cauchemez et al., 2009).

School closures can be pre-emptive (i.e., before an impending outbreak) or reactive (i.e., closure during the pandemic due to staff illness). Reactive closures may occur too late in an outbreak to have any meaningful benefit (Davis et al., 2015), whereas proactive closures can slow the spread of infection (House et al., 2011; Kawaguchi et al., 2009; Wu et al., 2010). There has been a concern that students dismissed from schools may congregate elsewhere, thereby undermining efforts aimed at social distancing to mitigate disease transmission. However, research suggests that school closure decreases the number of social contacts among school children (Aiello et al., 2010).

Potential adverse effects of school closure include (1) loss of access to school nutrition programs (breakfast and lunch) for the underprivileged, (2) lack of child-care for low-income working parents, (3) income loss if parents have to stay home to look after their children, and (4) disrupted learning (Berkman, 2008). These concerns are moot if schools are simply unable to remain open during a pandemic because of illness-related staff absenteeism. Nevertheless, if schools must be closed then it is important to plan to mitigate the negative effects on students and their caregivers.

As for social distancing in general, social isolation is a potential adverse effect (Abeysinghe & White, 2010). Fortunately, however, people can gain significant social contact and social support from social media (e.g., Facebook, Twitter, Snapchat) (Trepte & Scharkow, 2017). Therefore, physical isolation due to social distancing need not necessarily lead to a significant erosion of social contact and social support.

The economic hardship associated with social distancing is a more important problem. About 40% of American workers in the private sector do not have paid sick leave (Levi et al., 2010) and therefore suffer economic hardship during work closure. This disproportionately affects women, low wage-earners, and part-time workers (US Congress Joint Economic Committee, 2010). People have also expressed concerns about the closure of places of worship during pandemics, citing the need for shared support and worship during times of crisis (Baum, Jacobson, & Goold, 2009; Schoch-Spana, 2004). For these and other reasons discussed later in this volume, many people fail to adhere to social distancing recommendations during a pandemic. During the 2009 Swine flu pandemic, for example, a study of faculty and students at the University of Delaware revealed that very few people (6-9%) with acute respiratory infection actually stayed home when ill, and many sick people (45%) attended social events even though they were contagious (Mitchell et al., 2011). A multinational study during the same pandemic found that many respondents from the UK and US

(79% and 44%, respectively) made no effort to avoid being near someone who had influenza-like symptoms (SteelFisher et al., 2012). Most respondents (89% and 72%) made no attempt to avoid crowded public places such as shopping centers or sporting events.

Although sick people may be advised to remain home during a pandemic, forced isolation and quarantine may be ineffective and impractical (WHO Writing Group, 2006). It has been well documented that people often refuse to adhere to quarantine guidelines (e.g., BBC News, 2003; Georges-Courbot, Leroy, & Zeller, 2002). Nonadherence to social distancing occurs even during highly lethal outbreaks. During an outbreak of Ebola virus disease in Africa, some family members concealed sick relatives at home rather than sending them to quarantine facilities (Shultz et al., 2015). Another striking example of defiance of quarantine laws was described during the Bubonic Plague of 1630:

> Health monitors were hired to patrol the streets watching for plague victims. These monitors sent the plague victims to the pesthouses [plague houses], had their belongings burned and their homes disinfected and boarded up; very often with other family members still inside. However, the people fought back by withholding reporting plague cases to the authorities, risking *strappado*; a punishment of having their hands bound behind their backs, and then being hung by the wrists. People became adept at hiding their sick relatives or even co-workers, in the hope that the victim may be spared the pesthouse. (Staiano, 2008, p. 142)

Social distancing also can be undermined by competing government interests. Governments sometimes attempt to deny the presence of infection in an attempt to avoid the damaging effects that infectious outbreaks have on foreign trade and on public anxiety. Moscow, for example, denied the existence of Bubonic Plague in 1770, despite 4,000 deaths that year, in an attempt to maintain foreign trade (Staiano, 2008). During the 2003 SARS outbreak, health officials in China knew about the outbreak well before it was publicly acknowledged (Cheng, 2004). Attempts to downplay the danger were also evident during the Spanish flu. Governmental and health authorities attempted to downplay the prevalence and seriousness of infection in an attempt to quell public anxiety. To illustrate, in a 1918 memorandum sent from the Canadian Department of Militia and Defence in Ottawa to the assistant director of medical services in Toronto, it was advised that:

> Every effort must be made to control alarm, not only among the troops but among the public and the Press. The daily publication of statistics is very undesirable. (Pettigrew, 1983, p. 15)

Conclusion

Contemporary methods for managing pandemics include risk communication, vaccines and antiviral medication, hygiene practices, and social distancing. Psychological factors play an essential role in the success or failure of each of these methods. Psychological factors are important in the development of risk communication messages and such factors determine the impact of such messages. Psychological factors also play a vital role in adherence to vaccines, hygiene, and social distancing. Nonadherence is a notorious problem. A deeper understanding of the psychology of pandemics is needed to understand why adherence to infection management programs can be so poor and how it might be improved.

CHAPTER 3

PSYCHOLOGICAL REACTIONS TO PANDEMICS

Importance of Psychological Factors

Contemporary methods for managing pandemics are largely behavioral or educational interventions—that is, vaccination adherence programs, hygienic practices, and social distancing—in which psychological factors play a vital role. Excessive emotional distress associated with threatened or actual infection is a further issue of clinical and public health significance. Psychological factors are also relevant for understanding and addressing the socially disruptive behavioral patterns that can arise as a result of widespread, serious infection.

Emotional Reactions to Threats of Harm, Loss, and Change

Most people are resilient to stress, and many survivors of highly stressful events will likely emerge psychologically unscathed (Shultz et al., 2008; Taylor, 2017). However, during the next pandemic, many people will become fearful, some intensely so. The psychological "footprint" will likely be larger than the medical "footprint" (Shultz et al., 2008). That is, the psychological effects of the next pandemic will likely be more pronounced, more widespread, and longer-lasting than the purely somatic effects of infection. This was seen during the 2014-2015 Ebola outbreak in West Africa, in which the "epidemic of fear" was worse than the epidemic itself in terms of the number of people affected (Desclaux, Diop, & Doyon, 2017). Excessive public fear of Ebola even arose in the United States even though there was little or no risk of contagion (Kilgo, Yoo, & Johnson, 2018; Parmet & Sinha, 2017). A similar situation arose during the 2003 SARS outbreak. Although SARS was dangerous to the elderly and medically frail (Lee, 2014), the psychological impact of SARS was far greater than the medical impact in terms of the number of people affected and the duration for which they were affected (Cheng, 2004; Washer, 2004). For some people, the psychological effects of SARS persisted long after they had recovered from the virus, as discussed below.

Although many people will probably experience emotional distress during the next pandemic, the picture will be more complex. People differ in how they react to psychosocial stressors such as the threat of, or an actual occurrence of, a pandemic. Reactions can be diverse, ranging from fear to indifference to fatalism (Honingsbaum, 2009; Pettigrew, 1983; Wheaton, Abramowitz, Berman, Fabricant, & Olatunji, 2012). At one end of the spectrum, some people frankly disregard or deny the risks, and fail to engage in recommended health behaviors such as vaccination, hygiene practices, and social distancing. At the other end of the spectrum, many people react with intense anxiety or fear. A moderate level of fear or anxiety can motivate people to cope with health threats, but severe distress can be debilitating.

Fear of an impending pandemic can precede any actual pandemic and may have to be dealt with in addition to managing the pandemic itself (van den Bulck & Custers, 2009). The surge of patients on hospitals can occur even when an outbreak is only a rumor. During the 2009 Swine flu pandemic, for example, consider a study conducted in Utah. At a time when there was heightened public concern about influenza but little disease prevalence in Utah, emergency room departments experienced substantial surges in patient volumes, with the volumes comparable to the increases experienced when the disease actually reached the state (McDonnell, Nelson, & Schunk, 2012). Most of the surge was due to pediatric visits. Young children frequently contract diseases with flu-like features (e.g., fever, cough, congestion), which were likely misinterpreted by their parents as possible signs of Swine flu.

Anxiety and fear become even more prevalent when the pandemic actually arrives. During the early stages of the 2009 Swine flu pandemic, for example, 24% of a UK community sample reported significant anxiety about the outbreak (Rubin, Amlôt, Page, & Wessely, 2009). In a survey of American college students during the early stages of the same pandemic, most (83%) reported at least some degree of anxiety about becoming infected (Kanadiya & Sallar, 2011). Some people may develop excessive fears of death and disability, while others may express fears of being shunned by others if they were to become ill (Cheng, Wong, Tsang, & Wong, 2004). Some people may become so anxious that they experience clinically significant levels of distress, avoidance, and functional impairment, to a level that they may require treatment for their emotional disorder (Wheaton et al., 2012).

Repetitive checking and reassurance seeking can occur in response to the threat of infection (Taylor & Asmundson, 2004). During the early stages of the Swine flu pandemic, a British government online diagnostic website was unable to keep up with the demand for information, with the site crashing as thousands of people simultaneously tried to access the website (Bowcott & Carrell, 2009). Excessive (medically unnecessary) checking and reassurance seeking are characteristic features of people who are unduly worried about their health (Taylor & Asmundson, 2017). Such behaviors can place a significant burden on the healthcare system (Tyrer & Tyrer, 2018).

People who are highly anxious about being infected typically go to great lengths to protect themselves. This may involve avoidance of infection-related stimuli, including people, places, and things associated with disease. People may refuse to go to work for fear of coming in contact with infected others. During the Spanish flu pandemic, there were reports of sick, bedridden people starving to death because they were avoided by others (Barry, 2009). Avoidance or fearful removal of perceived sources of infection can even extend to animals. During the 2003 SARS outbreak in China there were widespread reports of household dogs and cats being abandoned, euthanized, or sometimes brutally killed (e.g., beaten to death), because of fear that the animals might be carrying the SARS virus (Epstein, 2003).

People may go to great lengths to "decontaminate" perceived sources of infection or to remove perceived contaminants from themselves. This may involve behaviors that are more extreme than mere handwashing. During the SARS outbreak, one woman in Beijing microwaved banknotes that she had acquired from a bank, fearing that the notes were infected. The outcome was predictable; the money burst into flames and was incinerated (Cheng, 2004). People may engage in all kinds of protective or safety behaviors. For example, some people have been getting vaccinated twice in one flu season (i.e., receiving trivalent and quadrivalent vaccines) when only one vaccination would suffice (Saxena, 2018).

Mental disorders can be triggered or exacerbated by pandemic-related stressors, including mood disorders, anxiety disorders, and posttraumatic stress disorder (PTSD) (Shultz et al., 2015; Wu, Chan, & Ma, 2005). PTSD can be triggered by pandemic-related stressors such as exposure to widespread mortality, and including the deaths of loved ones (Shultz et al., 2008; Taylor, 2017). Although there are few data on the incidence of PTSD from influenza pandemics, anecdotal reports suggest that some survivors had repetitive, vivid, detailed recollections of pandemic-related stressors, suggestive of PTSD reexperiencing symptoms. Some of these occurred decades after the event, as suggested by the following account from a 96-year-old woman who described her repetitive, intrusive recollections of the funeral of her mother, father, and brother in Britain during the 1918 Spanish flu pandemic.

> It's like a film in my head. There were the black horses with the plumes made from ostrich feathers, then the gun carriage with my dad's coffin covered with the union flag. My mother's coffin was in a big glass hearse with Noel's coffin under the driver's seat. (Honigsbaum, 2009, p. 104)

Depression or severe grief can occur in people who have lost loved ones during a pandemic. As recalled by one Spanish flu survivor, "Every day there was someone we knew in the obituary columns" (Pettigrew, 1983, p. 16). Severe guilt may occur if a person believes they should have saved loved ones or believes they were somehow responsible for the spread of disease (Taylor, 2017).

As a pandemic unfolds, some people adapt to the threat and become less anxious. However, in some cases the psychological effects can be severe and long-lasting. Research on the SARS outbreak shows that the psychological effects are not always short-lived, and that emotional reactions can be severe and persistent.

SARS arose from a novel strain of coronavirus, causing flu-like symptoms with prominent respiratory distress, which in many cases led to pneumonia. When SARS emerged in 2002-2003, little was known about its course or optimal management. Worldwide, SARS infected over 8,000 people and about 10% died (WHO, 2004). SARS has been described as a mental health catastrophe (Gardner & Moallef, 2015) because of widespread psychopathology associated with the disease. Various types of SARS-related fears predominated, including fear for survival and fear of infecting others, and some patients developed symptoms of PTSD. To illustrate the latter, a longitudinal (2-46 month) study found that 44% of SARS patients developed PTSD (Hong et al., 2009). In another survey of Beijing hospital workers during the SARS outbreak, about 10% developed PTSD symptoms (Wu et al., 2009). Respondents who had been quarantined, worked at high-risk sites such as SARS wards, or had friends or close relatives who contracted SARS, were 2-3 times more likely to have PTSD symptoms than people without these exposures (Wu et al., 2009). Quarantine can be distressing for many people, with some experiencing anxiety for their safety or anger about being involuntarily confined.

For many SARS patients, psychological distress, including PTSD symptoms, persisted well after the infection had been treated, in some cases for years after patients had recovered from the physical effects of the SARS virus (Gardner & Moallef, 2015). What made SARS especially distressing was that it was (1) a novel infection with an unknown course and treatment, (2) infection was managed with social isolation, and (3) there were fears of spreading this poorly understood infection to others (Maunder et al., 2006). These issues raise concerns about the long-term psychological consequences of the next pandemic.

SARS was also associated with psychotic symptoms during the acute and early recovery phases (Gardner & Moallef, 2015). These symptoms were linked to steroid treatments, which are used to manage the cytokine release syndrome ("cytokine storm") that can arise from severe infections (Channappanavar & Perlman, 2017). The occurrence of SARS-related psychosis raises concerns that such symptoms might occur during the next pandemic. Indeed, severe influenza can be associated with the cytokine release syndrome (Liu, Zhou, & Yang, 2016), which would be managed with steroids, with short-term psychosis being a potential adverse effect. Psychosis is not simply distressing to the individual; terrifying psychotic experiences can be traumatizing, leading to, or exacerbating, symptoms of PTSD (Taylor, 2017).

It is important to understand what leads people to become excessively distressed during outbreaks of severe infectious disease. This can help predict who is likely to need psychological services when the next pandemic arises. Understanding the causes of excessive distress can also be useful in developing optimal psychological treatments for affected individuals. There are various kinds of risk factors, including personality factors discussed in Chapter 5.

The Desperate Pursuit of Quack Cures and Folk Remedies

When faced with danger, such as a serious health threat, people can be highly irrational in their decision making (Ariely, 2014). If the next pandemic proves to be highly lethal and refractory to available vaccines and antiviral medications, people desperate to protect themselves and loved ones will increasingly turn to quack cures and dubious folk remedies. There is a long history of such nostrums for influenza, including wearing necklaces of garlic, inhaling carbolic acid vapors, and consuming pine tar (Bristow, 2012; Petrovska & Cekovska, 2010; Simpson, 1985). Similarly, during the 2003 SARS outbreak, there were numerous folk remedies, all of which were ineffective. These included diets of turnips, vinegar, kimchee, or spicy foods, and even smoking cigarettes (Cheng, 2004).

During the Spanish flu of 1918, folk remedies included cotton bags containing camphor, worn on a cord around the neck (Arnold, 2018b). There were all sorts of recipes for poultices. A poultice is a soft, usually heated, moist mass of material, usually consisting of plant material or flour, that is placed on the body (e.g., on the chest) to relieve soreness or inflammation, and held in place with a cloth.

> Some people put their faith in violet-leaf tea, goose-grease poultices, garlic buds, castor oil, salt water snuffed up the nose, or hot coals sprinkled with sulphur or brown sugar and carried through the house accompanied by clouds of billowing smoke. ... There were many theories about the most effective mixtures for chest poultices: bran, as hot as you could stand; lard mixed with camphor and chloroform; and a half-and-half mix of lard and turpentine. (Pettigrew, 1983, p. 110)

In one instance a Canadian man drank hydrogen peroxide in the hope of keeping himself safe from the Spanish flu:

> Having heard that hydrogen peroxide was an effective germ-killer, [he] thought he would take extra precautions, so he bought a bottle of the liquid and drank as much of it as he could. Frothing and bubbling, he was rushed to the infirmary and luckily survived the drastic self-medication. Fortunately, too, he recovered from the influenza he caught a week later despite the peroxide. (Pettigrew, 1983, p. 115)

During pandemics, people may engage in all kinds of superstitious behaviors in the hope of keeping themselves or their loved ones safe. Here is another Canadian example from the Spanish flu pandemic:

> George H. Biddle, a Vancouver glazier and window washer who was in constant contact with the public, and whose family was down with the 'flu, believed he kept himself safe by sprinkling a bit of powdered sulphur into his shoes every morning before leaving the house. (Pettigrew, 1983, p. 114)

As the Spanish flu spread, many manufacturers and retailers were quick to turn it to their advantage (Pettigrew, 1983). Newspapers were filled with advertisements for quack remedies, including mint lozenges to be sucked whenever the person entered a crowded space (Arnold, 2018a). Patent medicines, likely no better than placebos, were advertised with wild claims of efficacy. Drug stores ran out of *Vick's VapoRub* and other balms. Even bicycle dealers attempted to exploit the pandemic for economic gain. During the Spanish flu pandemic, a Toronto newspaper ran the following advertisement:

> Get away from the stuffy, overcrowded street cars, with their danger of contagion. Ride a bicycle through the pure, fresh air. With an easy-running, long-lasting C.C.M. Bicycle, cycling will be a pleasure as well as a benefit. (Pettigrew, 1983, p. 113).

The situation is no different in recent times concerning quackery and folk remedies. During the 2003 SARS outbreak, there were reports from China, an officially atheist country, that some people had hired sorcerers, lit firecrackers, burned fake money, and practiced other magical rituals to protect themselves (Lee, 2014). A rumor spread about a miraculous child who could talk at birth and prophesied that green bean soup would prevent infection. This led to a sharp increase in the sale of mung beans (Lee, 2014).

Quack cures and folk remedies are widely available in stores and readily offered on the Internet. People may try to cope with the threat of infection by taking large doses of vitamins or herbal supplements in the hope that this will somehow boost their immune system (Lee, 2014). Some anti-vaccination conspiracy theorists claim that large doses of vitamin C are a cure-all (Pilkington & Glenza, 2019). Even contemporary pharmacies are stocked with quack remedies for treating influenza. To illustrate, Oscillococcinum® is widely sold in Western pharmacies and touted by the manufacturer as a homeopathic remedy for shortening the duration of flu symptoms (Lowrie, 2019). There is no evidence that Oscillococcinum works, and indeed no reason to expect it to work (Mathie, Frye, & Fisher, 2015). Oscillococcinum pills are made by taking extracts from the heart and liver of ducks, and then diluting the extracts until virtually no trace remains. Such homeopathic remedies have no benefits beyond placebo effects (Antonelli & Donelli, 2018; Ernst, 2010).

What motivates people to seek out dubious or frankly bogus treatments? Diverse motivations are likely to be at play, including imitation, conformity, desperation, and indiscriminate reliance on authority figures. According to one survivor of the Spanish flu pandemic:

> My mother used goose grease and turpentine mixed like a salve, sometimes she made a poultice out of it. I think it really helped. She told me it did, so I had to believe it. (Pettigrew, 1983, p. 120)

People may try to hedge their bets by pursuing both mainstream and fringe medicine. Some people apply salves or consume elixirs "just to be one the safe side," as amply illustrated by accounts from the Spanish flu, such as the following.

> Alongside over-the-counter products, frightened families also turned to folk remedies, traditional and reassuring cures familiar to their heritage, whether this be onions, asafetida (a fetid-smelling herb historically used for chest complaints), or opium. As the mortality rates soared, so too did the willingness to try something, anything, to save themselves and their loved ones from a horrible death. (Arnold, 2018a, p. 1)

Factors that play a role in anxiety proneness also likely play a role in motivating the pursuit of quack cures. People who are prone to excessive worry or anxiety, as discussed later in this volume, are likely to desperately try a range of nostrums, no matter how dubious, to avoid becoming infected. We can expect to see a rise of quack cures, folk remedies, and superstitious health-related behaviors during the next pandemic.

Civil Unrest, Rioting, and Mass Panic

Mass panic is a group phenomenon in which intensely frightened people think only of themselves, causing harm to others as they struggle to save themselves (Shultz et al., 2008). Mass panic and widespread antisocial behavior, such as rioting, looting, and the destruction of property, sometimes but not usually occur during pandemics (Shultz et al., 2008). Affiliative, supportive, prosocial behaviors are more common, where widespread sickness and debility evoke acts of mutual aid among members of a community in crisis (Dezecache, 2015; Pettigrew, 1983; Schoch-Spana, 2004). But even then, people are cautious and fearful of helping others.

> Often it was an agonizing decision: go to the aid of friends and relatives, perhaps imperiling the safety of their own families, or keep away? The moral decision to close the doors was frequently as difficult as that to go out and help. (Pettigrew, 1983, p. 88)

Despite the occurrence of prosocial acts, riots have sometimes erupted during times of pandemic and other infectious disease outbreaks (Cohn, 2010). During the Bubonic Plague in 1587, for example, a doctor in Rome's principal hospital in Santo Spirito opined that "Beyond all doubt, plague gives rise to fights among the populace, sedition, and revolt" (Cohn, 2010, p. 265). Indeed, historians have long noted the rise of factional violence, criminality, and rioting during times of plague (Cohn, 2010). This included looting and the pilfering of possessions from the bodies of the deceased and the homes of plague victims.

There are numerous examples, both historical and contemporary, in which groups of citizens clashed violently with health authorities, fearing that the authorities were harming rather than helping them. Here are some examples:

> In September 2014, a team of eight health workers and journalists disappeared shortly after arriving in the southern Guinean village of Wome [in Africa], not far from the place where the Ebola outbreak first erupted eight months earlier... They had come to teach Wome's villagers how to protect themselves against Ebola. But instead of welcoming their helpers, the villagers attacked them with stones, clubs, and machetes, believing that the workers to be spreaders of the disease. The attackers then slit the visitors' throats and dumped the bodies in the village cistern where they were discovered three days later. (Quick, 2018, p. 149)

> Villagers [in China] protesting the local government's SARS policy in Zhejiang province stormed local offices, breaking windows and office furniture and assaulting officials. (Lee, 2014, p. 25)

> In 1894, people in a poor south-side community in Milwaukee, Wisconsin, attacked police and ambulances during a city-wide smallpox outbreak. ... Mobs wielded household items from baseball bats to potato mashers, anything that would serve as weapons. People tossed pots of scalding water on the horses pulling the ambulances. Rioting went on for a month. Citizens were so fearful of health authorities that they hid the sick, which naturally increased the rates of infection within households. (Quick, 2018, p. 150).

Economic hardship can also lead to civil unrest during pandemics. During the 1575-1578 Bubonic Plague outbreak in Venice, cloth merchants employed two-thirds of the city's workforce. When plague broke out, merchants closed their shops and some fled to the countryside, thereby depriving workers and artisans of their livelihood. The closure of their shops led to widespread unemployment. This, in turn, led to fights for resources, including fights over the possessions of the dead (Cohn, 2010).

There have also been many documented cases of panic buying. During an outbreak of Avian flu, there was panic buying of food, disinfectants, and the antiviral medication oseltamivir (Tamiflu) (Cheng, 2004, 2005). In Baltimore during the Spanish flu pandemic, "customers ravaged drug stores in search of products to prevent influenza and relieve symptoms" (Schoch-Spana, 2004, p. 45). In Winnipeg, Canada, during the same pandemic Dr. F. T. Cadham of the Canadian Army Medical Corps, was running tests on an experimental vaccine. "Dr. Cadham had to have a police escort as he drove from his home to his office, so anxious were people to get the vaccine" (Pettigrew, 1983, p. 20). There was also panic buying and rioting during the 1968 Hong Kong flu pandemic (Wilson et al., 2009). During that pandemic, in the city of Guangzhou, China, there was a lack of medication due to the public's buying up and hoarding of pharmacy supplies, along with rioting and looting of food from restaurants and grocery stores (Wilson, Iannarone, & Wang, 2009).

Rioting and civil protests can occur when it is widely believed that some group, particularly a group in the position of authority, is somehow to blame (Tufekci & Freelon, 2013). In the case of pandemics or other outbreaks, riots can be sparked by grievances against, or perceived injustices from, health authorities. Bubonic plague outbreaks led to rioting in India in the 1890s, arising from rumors that the British were complicit in spreading the disease (Chandavarkar, 1992). For similar reasons, cholera outbreaks in Europe in the 1830s led to rioting.

> Popular opinion did not accept that cholera was a hitherto unknown disease, but considered instead that an attempt was being made to reduce the numbers of the poor by poisoning them. Riots, massacres and the destruction of property took place across Russia, swept through the Habsburg empire, broke out in Konigsberg, Stettin and Memel in 1831 and spread to Britain the next year. (Evans, 1992, p. 158)

Although many people are reluctant to seek vaccination, as discussed elsewhere in this volume, many other people ardently seek vaccination against seasonal influenza. Civil unrest and protests can occur when people become frustrated by the lack of availability of vaccines. For example, in the US in the winter of 2004-2005, there was a shortage of seasonal influenza vaccine due to production problems at one of the manufacturing plants.

> As the shortfall materialized, federal and state health officials tried to distribute the limited number of vaccine doses to individuals most at risk, such as the elderly and those with compromised immune systems. Nevertheless, there were incidents in which crowds of elderly and infirm people waited for hours at clinics and health centers for the vaccine, only to learn that there was none to be had. One New York City clinic actually called in the police to stop a riot by mostly elderly people. (Norkin, 2014)

Clearly, rioting is not an activity exclusively for young people. Although pandemic-related riots have been well-documented, some commentators have asked why riots don't happen more often (Newburn, 2016). The actions of crowds are notoriously difficult to forecast (Hoegh, Ferreira, & Leman, 2016). Social media and the 24-hour news cycle in which events are unfolded in real-time can play a role in rallying people toward social unrest (Hoegh et al., 2016; Tufekci & Freelon, 2013), especially because in times of crisis many people turn to social media for information and guidance (Devine, Boluk, & Devine, 2017). It is an open question as to the extent to which panic buying, rioting and other forms of civil dissent will occur during the next pandemic. Some risk analysts have advocated that we prepare for the worst.

> If the pandemic is severe, the hardest job won't be coping with the disease. It will be sustaining the flow of essential goods and services, and maintaining civil order. ... Even though we hope riots, panics and other sorts of civil disorder will not be common, it is important to be on guard. (Sandman, 2009, p. 323)

In a 2005 report the WHO predicted that widespread panic could occur during the next pandemic if supplies of antiviral drugs are severely limited or ineffective and a suitable vaccine is not yet available (WHO, 2005). Shultz and colleagues (2008) pointed out that food shortages could lead to widespread panic and civil disruption could occur during the next pandemic:

> The possibility of extreme food shortages due to hoarding, border closures, and the rapid evaporation of just-in-time inventories (without options for re-supply) may create some of the most grievous consequences of a global pandemic. Much of the world population is now living in urban areas, completely dependent upon food and essential supplies that are produced elsewhere and must be continuously transported to urban markets. Food shortages may create chaos and completely upend public health measures intended to keep people apart to minimize infection risks. The imperative of seeking food and vital supplies could place many at risk for influenza infection. (Shultz et al., 2008, p. 222).

During the next pandemic, truck drivers and other food service delivery agents may refuse to enter infected cities, thereby leading the inhabitants to either starve or flee. Indeed, something similar happened during the Bubonic Plague, in which farmers refused to deliver their produce to infected cities (Cohn, 2010).

There are several other plausible scenarios in which, during the next pandemic, panic and civil unrest could arise because of the spread of unfounded rumors via social media (Walker, 2016):

- An unfounded rumor sends tens of thousands of citizens to local pharmacies in dozens of major cities, overwhelming them and triggering riots or looting as panicked people demand a drug the stores don't carry or that is irrelevant to the pandemic disease.
- In cities that serve as major airport hubs, a handful of cases of a disease are filmed and sensationalized, generating enough fear to cause tens of thousands of people to flee those cities and effectively cripple them. Business, industry, and air travel would quickly become disrupted.
- An unfounded rumor persuades enough health workers not to show up to the leading hospitals in a handful of major cities, effectively shutting them down. A chain reaction ensues whereby hundreds of other hospitals are quickly inundated and then overwhelmed.

Immunologically Induced Psychological Reactions

So far, we have focused mainly on emotional reactions that occur in people who have not yet been infected. There is another class of psychological reactions that are the direct physiological consequence of infection. People infected by viral or bacterial agents may experience a syndrome called sickness behavior (Dantzer, O'Connor, Freund, Johnson, & Kelley, 2008). Symptoms include nausea, fatigue, sleep disturbance, depression, irritability, and mild cognitive impairment (problems with memory and attention). Sickness behavior is not simply a reaction to the discomfort of fever; sickness behavior and fever are distinguishable reactions to infection (Corrard et al., 2017). Sickness behavior is triggered by proinflammatory cytokines such as tumor necrosis factor-α, interleukin-6, and interleukin-1β (Shattuck & Muehlenbein, 2016). Immune reactions can involve neuroinflammation, which may lead to sickness behavior (Dantzer, 2009; Zhu, Levasseur, Michaelis, Burfeind, & Marks, 2016).

Little is known about whether some people are especially prone to sickness behavior, although it has been speculated that people with a predisposition to emotional disorders may be particularly vulnerable (Dantzer, 2009). Reactions suggestive of sickness behavior have been observed during pandemics (e.g., Honigsbaum, 2014), although it can be difficult to determine whether emotional reactions (e.g., irritability, depression) are due to an immune response (sickness behavior) or whether they are reactions to psychosocial stressors (e.g., physical hardships due to food shortages, crowding at hospitals, or loss of loved ones). Treatments for emotional disorders—including drugs such as selective serotonin reuptake inhibitors and cognitive-behavior therapy (CBT)—can be efficacious even if, say, depression is part of the sickness behavior syndrome (Dantzer, 2009).

Interactions Between Stress and the Immune System

Decades of research in the field of psychoneuroimmunology have shown that negative emotions and stressful life events can lead to some degree of suppression of the immune system, thereby enhancing susceptibility to infection and dampening the beneficial effects of vaccines (Irwin & Slavich, 2017; Kiecolt-Glaser, 2009). To illustrate, a series of studies has shown that immune responses to viral and bacterial vaccines, including influenza vaccines, are delayed, substantially weakened, or shorter-lived in people who are distressed or exposed to stressors (Glaser & Kiecolt-Glaser, 2005; Kiecolt-Glaser, 2009). These effects tend to be greatest in people who are prone to experience frequent negative moods (i.e., negative emotionality; see Chapter 5) (Phillips, Carroll, Burns, & Drayson, 2005). The mechanisms of these effects are still under investigation, although stressors and negative emotions have been found to influence the production of lymphocytes and proinflammatory cytokines (Irwin & Slavich, 2017; Kiecolt-Glaser, 2009).

Psychoneuroimmunology research suggests that pandemic-related stressors may compromise the immune system, thereby making people more vulnerable to infection. People who are prone to frequently experience intense anxiety or other negative emotions (see Chapter 5), compared to people who experience these emotions less frequently and less intensely, may be more susceptible to pandemic influenza infection, and may benefit less from vaccination. But even if pandemic-related stress and distress do significantly dampen the immune system, psychological interventions such as CBT (see Chapter 11) can reduce a person's stress proneness and negative emotions, thereby offsetting any stress-related immunosuppression (Moraes, Miranda, Loures, Mainieri, & Mármora, 2017).

Conclusion

The patterns of psychological reactions to pandemics are complex. Whereas some people are resilient to stress, other individuals become highly distressed when confronted with threatening events such as pandemic infection. Thus, people vary widely in their reactions to threatened or actual pandemics. Some react with indifference or resignation while others become highly fearful or anxious, and some develop emotional disorders such as PTSD. Some people recover from these emotional problems once the pandemic threat passes, while other people have enduring emotional reactions. Social disruptive behaviors such as rioting can also occur under particular circumstances, although prosocial behaviors appear to be more common during times of pandemic. Immune reactions may explain some of the emotional responses in infected people but these fail to account for widespread fear and social disruption in people who have not yet been infected. To better understand the reasons behind these diverse psychological reactions it is important to understand their motivational roots and vulnerability factors. These are the topics of the following chapters.

CHAPTER 4

PERSONALITY TRAITS AS EMOTIONAL VULNERABILITY FACTORS

Vulnerability to Emotional Distress

There is no single theory for understanding the various emotional and other reactions to pandemics. There are, however, several mutually complementary domains of theory and research that are relevant: (1) Research on particular personality traits as vulnerability factors for experiencing distress in response to a range of stressors; (2) cognitive-behavioral models of health anxiety; (3) the concept of the behavioral immune system, which focuses specifically on motivational responses to perceived risk of infection; (4) analyses of social psychological factors in the spreading of fear, distress, and disease; (5) research on vaccination attitudes; and (6) studies on risk communication. The first domain is discussed in this chapter. The others are covered in later chapters.

Personality Traits

Personality refers to a constellation of traits possessed by a person that define how she or he tends to think, feel, and behave across various situations. The traits are dimensional in that a person may possess varying degrees of a given trait. People with high scores on the trait of extraversion, for example, tend to be highly outgoing and sociable. People scoring low on this trait are less likely to be interested in socializing.

Several personality traits have been linked to the proneness to experience negative emotions in response to stressors. These traits are interrelated and transdiagnostic in that they are associated with a range of emotional problems (Kring & Sloan, 2010; Norton & Paulus, 2017). Theoretically, people scoring high on one or more on scales measuring these traits, compared to people with low scores, are most likely to become distressed in response to a wide range of threatening events, including the threat of an influenza pandemic. The following is a review of relevant traits, including those traits that have been investigated in relation to infectious outbreaks and appear most promising for understanding psychological reactions to future pandemics. Such traits can be measured by any of several empirically validated questionnaires (e.g., Buhr & Dugas, 2002; Cloninger, 1994; Frost & Steketee, 2002; Spielberger, 1979; Taylor et al., 2007; Watson & O'Hara, 2017).

Negative Emotionality

Negative emotionality, also known as neuroticism, is the general tendency to become easily distressed by aversive stimuli. People scoring high on this trait tend to frequently experience aversive emotions such as anxiety, irritability, and depression in response to stressors (Costa & McCrae, 1987). Negative emotionality is a risk factor for various kinds of mood and anxiety disorders (Watson & O'Hara, 2017). Negative emotionality is also associated with anxiety about one's general health (Asmundson, Taylor, & Cox, 2001; Boelen & Carleton, 2012; Fergus, Bardeen, & Orcutt, 2015; van Dijk et al., 2016). This is because people scoring high on negative emotionality tend to misinterpret bodily sensations as indications of serious disease (Ferguson, 2000). Therefore, it is not surprising that the severity of a person's negative emotionality predicts their likelihood of becoming distressed by the threat of infection. During the 2003 SARS epidemic, for example, negative emotionality predicted the level of distress experienced by HCWs who were responsible for caring for patients with suspected SARS (Lu, Shu, Chang, & Lung, 2006). A study of college students similarly found that negative emotionality predicted the level of distress in response to the threat of Avian flu infection (Smith, Kay, Hoyt, & Bernard, 2009). People with high levels of negative emotionality are also less likely to be satisfied with their interactions with their doctors (Ferguson, 2000), which could be a factor in persistently seeking medical reassurance or "doctor shopping" (see Chapter 5).

Trait Anxiety and Harm Avoidance

Negative emotionality is a higher-order trait that is made up of several narrower traits, including two conceptually overlapping traits: Trait anxiety and harm avoidance. Trait anxiety is the proneness to experience anxiety. People scoring high on trait anxiety tend to view the world as dangerous and threatening (Spielberger, 1979). Harm avoidance refers to the tendency to avoid potential risk. People with high levels of harm avoidance tend to be fearful and worry excessively (Cloninger, 1994). Harm avoidance and trait anxiety are both correlated with anxiety disorders, mood disorders, obsessive-compulsive disorder, somatoform disorders, and with health anxiety (e.g., Ecker, Kupfer, & Gönner, 2014; Huang et al., 2016; Melli, Chiorri, Carraresi, Stopani, & Bulli, 2015). Trait anxiety also predicted the level of SARS-related anxiety during the SARS outbreak (Cheng & Cheung, 2005).

Overestimation of Threat

Just as negative emotionality is made up of numerous narrower traits, so too is trait anxiety. Trait anxiety is composed of various lower-order traits including a trait known as the overestimation of threat. People who score high on the overestimation of threat tend to overestimate the cost ("badness") and probability (likelihood) of aversive events, and see themselves as being especially vulnerable to threats (Frost & Steketee, 2002; Moritz & Pohl, 2009). People scoring high on the overestimation of threat are likely to endorse statements such as the following: "I believe that the world is a dangerous place," "Bad things are more likely to happen to me than to other people," and "Small things always seem to turn into big ones in my life" (Frost & Steketee, 2002). The overestimation of threat is associated with a range of clinical conditions, particularly anxiety disorders and obsessive-compulsive disorder (Frost & Steketee, 2002; Green & Teachman, 2013; Obsessive-Compulsive Cognitions Working Group, 2005). Studies have shown that the overestimation of threat predicts anxiety in response to outbreaks of SARS, Swine flu, Avian flu, and Ebola virus disease (e.g., Bish & Michie, 2010; Blakey, Reuman, Jacoby, & Abramowitz, 2015; Lau, Kim, Tsui, & Griffiths, 2008; Wheaton et al., 2012; Xie, Stone, Zheng, & Zhang, 2011). During the next pandemic, people who score high on the overestimation of threat are likely to become highly worried and anxious because their estimates of being harmed tend to be inflated compared to the estimates of people scoring lower on these traits.

Intolerance of Uncertainty

The intolerance of uncertainty is another facet or sub-trait of trait anxiety that can contribute to the tendency to experience anxiety and fear (McEvoy & Mahoney, 2013). People with high levels of intolerance of uncertainty have a strong desire for predictability and tend to strongly endorse statements such as "You should always look ahead to avoid surprises". When faced with important uncertainties, these people might feel paralyzed with indecision (Birrell, Meares, Wilkinson, & Freeston, 2011). They often endorse statements such as "The smallest doubt stops me from acting". Such people are unable to act or make decisions either because they worry they don't have all the information they need, or because they lack confidence in the soundness of their decisions. Such people tend to procrastinate about making important decisions.

A high degree of intolerance of uncertainty is associated with a range of disorders, including mood and anxiety disorders, obsessive-compulsive disorder, and other clinical conditions (Gentes & Ruscio, 2011; Rosser, 2018; Shihata, McEvoy, Mullan, & Carleton, 2016). Intolerance of uncertainty is associated with the tendency to worry excessively about a range of issues (Lauriola et al., 2018; Vander Haegen & Etienne, 2016), and is associated with health anxiety (Fergus et al., 2015; O'Bryan & McLeish, 2017; Shihata et al., 2016; Thibodeau et al., 2015).

People with high levels of intolerance of uncertainty try to reduce uncertainty by behaviors such as checking and reassurance-seeking (Dugas & Robichaud, 2007; Shihata et al., 2016). In the case of health-related uncertainty, this might involve repeatedly checking the Internet for medical information, and persistently seeking reassurance from doctors (Bottesi, Ghisi, Sica, & Freeston, 2017; Fergus, 2015; Lauriola et al., 2018; Norr, Albanese, Oglesby, Allan, & Schmidt, 2015).

During the next pandemic, the intolerance of uncertainty is likely to be a particularly important contributor to pandemic-related anxiety and distress. To understand the significance of this claim it is important to consider the range of uncertainties associated with pandemics.

Pandemics are associated with all kinds of uncertainties, such as the following: Uncertainty about getting infected, uncertainty about the seriousness of infection, uncertainty about whether the people around you are infected, uncertainty about whether objects or surfaces (e.g., money, doorknobs) are infected, uncertainty about the optimal type of treatment or protective measures, and uncertainty about whether a pandemic is truly over. Recall that pandemics come in waves, so the end of a wave of infection does not necessarily signal the end of the pandemic. There could be another wave, and the next wave could be more serious than the one before. The news media can fuel uncertainties with speculative articles about what "might" happen during an outbreak of infectious disease (Kilgo et al., 2018).

Such uncertainties are common sources of distress during pandemics (Taha, Matheson, Cronin, & Anisman, 2014). In the case of the 1918 Spanish flu pandemic, for example, it was not simply the high mortality rate that led to the fear of infection. The unpredictability of a swift, lethal infection was a major source of fear (Graves, 1969). As one survivor recalled, "We never knew where it would strike next" (Pettigrew, 1983, p. 13). The Spanish flu often struck with little or no warning, and some people, even seemingly healthy people, rapidly and unexpectedly perished. To illustrate:

> Two Woodstock, Ontario, girls, working in the town of Paris [in Ontario] shared a room at the YWCA. One evening when the epidemic was at its height they attended a lecture together and then returned to their room. In the morning Claire Hunter called to her friend, "Vera, I'm going downstairs to breakfast." There was no reply so she went ahead. After eating she went back upstairs to get her purse and called her roommate again. There was still no answer. "I pulled down the sheets. She was dead and cold. The doctor said she had died around two in the morning—the 'flu had got to her quick." (Pettigrew, 1983, p. 18)

During times of pandemic, people need to be able to tolerate or accept a certain degree of uncertainty. People who are unable or unwilling to accept uncertainty are likely to experience considerable distress. People with a high degree of intolerance of uncertainty tend to become highly anxious about the threat of infectious disease, especially if they perceive themselves as having limited control over the threat (Taha et al., 2014). To illustrate, during the 2009 Swine flu pandemic, people with a high degree of intolerance of uncertainty, compared to people with lower levels, were most likely to become anxious about contracting the virus (Taha et al., 2014). Such people tend to endorse statements such as "Even though there is a one in a million chance of me dying from the flu, so long as there is a chance, no matter how small, I'm worried that it could happen." During the same pandemic, the likelihood of seeking vaccination was greater in people with high levels of intolerance of uncertainty (Ashbaugh et al., 2013). However, during the next pandemic, the likelihood of seeking vaccination in people with high intolerance of uncertainty will likely depend on the availability of information about the safety of vaccines. If there are widely publicized doubts about vaccine safety, then it is likely that people who are intolerant of uncertainty will worry and procrastinate about whether to seek vaccination. Excessively high levels of intolerance of uncertainty can be effectively treated with CBT (Dugas & Robichaud, 2007).

Monitoring versus Blunting

People differ in the way they seek or avoid information about potential health threats. Some people tend to have a "monitoring" cognitive style, whereas other people tend to have a "blunting" style (Miller, 1989). Monitoring is characterized by collecting information and scanning for cues to health threats. Blunting involves distraction from, and minimizing of, threatening information (Miller, Fang, Diefenbach, & Bales, 2001). Monitoring and blunting can be measured with the Monitor-Blunter Style Scale (Miller, 1987), which is widely used in research on these cognitive styles.

Both styles have their shortcomings as coping strategies. Although blunting is generally associated with less health-related worry and distress, blunters are at risk for ignoring important health-related threats and failing to take precautionary measures (Miller, 1996). Monitors, compared to blunters, tend to perceive a given health threat as riskier and more dangerous and tend to be more vulnerable to everyday stress, especially when they perceive that their health is threatened (Miller et al., 2005). Monitors are more likely to engage in worrying than blunters, and this relationship between monitoring and worry was found to be independent of levels of trait anxiety (Davey, Hampton, Farrell, & Davidson, 1992; Miller, 1996).

During the next pandemic, monitors may experience significant levels of fear and anxiety, along with intrusive thoughts about threats, all of which may merit psychological treatment. Stress management training and other forms of CBT, as discussed later in this book, may be helpful (Miller, 1989). Monitors may benefit from interventions that help them learn how to monitor in a way that decreases the salience of threat and that instead focuses them on the positive and reassuring aspects of the situation, and in some cases on the things that they can *do* to effectively cope with and solve problems (Miller, 1996).

The distinction between monitoring and blunting also has implications for risk communication. Monitors can be motivated to engage in health behaviors by detailed information about risks and risk-reduction strategies (Kim & Choi, 2017). Blunters, in comparison, are likely to avoid such messages. Short, simple messages might be more effective for blunters (Kim & Choi, 2017). Monitors and blunters also appear to differ in how they respond to risk messages that involve logical versus emotional appeals (see Chapter 9).

Unrealistic Optimism Bias

Unlike the above-mentioned traits, which are associated with negative beliefs or expectations, the unrealistic optimism bias is associated with persistent and unrealistically positive beliefs about one's future (Taylor & Brown, 1988). Optimism—defined as the hope that something good is going to happen (Carver, Scheier, & Segerstrom, 2010)—can be a state variable or an enduring personality trait. Trait optimism, which is our focus here, is negatively correlated with negative emotionality, although the correlation is far from perfect. There is debate as to whether optimism is the opposite of pessimism or whether they are two different constructs (Kam & Meyer, 2012). Regardless of these theoretical debates, people scoring low on traits such as negative emotionality generally tend toward optimism.

Many people, although the precise prevalence is unknown, have an unrealistic optimism bias (Makridakis & Moleskis, 2015; Shepperd, Waters, Weinstein, & Klein, 2015). This is the strong tendency to believe that positive events are more likely to happen to themselves than to others, and that negative events are more likely to happen to other people than themselves (Weinstein, 1980). Such people tend to undervalue dangers such as diseases and other hardships, whose existence they accept but cannot believe will happen to themselves (Makridakis & Moleskis, 2015). People with a strong unrealistic optimism bias tend to see themselves as impervious to infection (Ji et al., 2004; Kim & Niederdeppe, 2013). During the SARS outbreak, for example, many people unrealistically thought that they were less susceptible to infection than the average person (Ji, Zhang, Usborne, & Guan, 2004).

In the event of a pandemic, the unrealistic optimism bias can have deleterious effects. It may lead people to underestimate their susceptibility to risk, thereby reducing attention to risk information and leading them to neglect to perform preventive health behaviors such as seeking vaccination (Kim & Niederdeppe, 2013). During the Swine flu outbreak in 2009, the unrealistic optimism bias was associated with lower intentions to perform hand washing and hand sanitization (Kim & Niederdeppe, 2013). The unrealistic optimism bias can be resistant to change in the face of disconfirming information (Sharot, Korn, & Dolan, 2011), although this is not invariably the case (Jefferson, Bortolotti, & Kuzmanovic, 2017).

Related to the unrealistic optimism bias is the sense of invulnerability. That is, the sense that one is unlikely to be affected by threats such as serious infectious disease. People with an inflated sense of invulnerability are (1) less likely to experience anxiety in response to stressful life events (Kleiman et al., 2017); (2) more likely to take up smoking or drug use (Hill, Duggan, & Lapsley, 2012; Morrell, Lapsley, & Halpern-Felsher, 2016; Ravert et al., 2009); (3) more likely to drink and drive (Chan, Wu, & Hung, 2010; Ravert et al., 2009); and (4) less likely to intend to seek vaccination, even for pandemics such as Swine flu (Taha et al., 2013).

During the next pandemic, people with strong unrealistic optimism bias or a strong sense of invulnerability will probably be less worried than other people and possibly more likely to spread infection by failing to seek vaccination and by neglecting to perform basic hygiene behaviors such as handwashing.

Other Personality Traits

Other traits are also correlated with pandemic-related anxiety. These include perfectionism, which has some similarities to intolerance of uncertainty in that it entails the search for solutions for avoiding danger. However, perfectionism is a trait that more broadly applies to achievement motivation (e.g., task performance) and other areas in life in which a person is judged against others (e.g., physical appearance) (Stoeber, 2018). For our aims, intolerance of uncertainty is more relevant than perfectionism for understanding the psychology of pandemics.

Another trait of potential relevance to pandemic-related anxiety is bodily vigilance, which is the tendency to notice or focus on anxiety-related sensations (Schmidt, Lerew, & Trakowski, 1997). A related concept is anxiety sensitivity, which is the fear of arousal- or anxiety-related bodily sensations (Taylor, 2019). People with high levels of anxiety sensitivity tend to be frightened of arousal- or anxiety-related bodily sensations (e.g., palpitations, shortness of breath) because they fear that the sensations will have harmful consequences. A person with a high level of anxiety sensitivity might hold the belief that "Palpitations lead to heart attacks" or that "If I become short of breath while I exercise, it means I could suffocate". Elevated anxiety sensitivity is associated with a range of different disorders, particularly panic disorder and other anxiety disorders (Taylor, 2019), and is correlated with fear or anxiety about becoming infected during a pandemic (Wheaton et al., 2012) and other outbreaks of infectious disease (Blakey et al., 2015). Conceptually, anxiety sensitivity (and body vigilance) overlaps with the concept of health anxiety, which is the topic of the following chapter. Both refer to the fear of bodily changes or sensations, and both can be treated with CBT.

Conclusion

Research indicates unrealistic optimism and related traits—including the sense of invulnerability and the blunting cognitive style—may be associated with low levels of pandemic-related anxiety and nonadherence to hygiene and other health recommendations. People who score highly on such traits would be particularly likely to spread contagion during a pandemic. Other personality traits, in comparison, are likely to be associated with high anxiety during the next pandemic. That is, various personality traits are vulnerability factors for high levels of emotional distress and therefore relevant to understanding pandemic-related worry and distress. A broad vulnerability factor is negative emotionality (neuroticism), which is composed of numerous narrower traits, including trait anxiety, the overestimation of threat, and intolerance of uncertainty. People with high scores on these traits are likely to become highly distressed when threatened with infection during a serious pandemic. These people, and people who have a monitoring coping style, are likely to exhibit worry or anxiety about their health. This has been termed *health anxiety*. We turn to the topic of health anxiety in the following chapter in order to gain a more detailed understanding of the thoughts, feelings, and behaviors that characterize health-anxious people.

CHAPTER 5

COGNITIVE-BEHAVIORAL MODELS OF HEALTH ANXIETY

What is Health Anxiety?

> Over the past few months I've been under a lot of stress because of my job. I haven't been feeling well. I feel achy all over and sick in my stomach. I don't sleep well. I sweat at night and feel tired all the time. I worry that I've got that bird flu everyone's been talking about. I went to the doctor but he wasn't any help. He said it was just nerves and told me to relax. I also have pain on my right side around my ribs. The doctor said it's just a strained muscle. I'm scared that he doesn't take me seriously. I couldn't stop worrying so I went to a walk-in clinic but the doctor told me the same thing as the other doctor. She said that I should try not to worry so much and gave me a prescription for pills to help me relax. I'm frightened of taking pills because I always get bad side effects. When I got home, I checked my symptoms on Google. That really terrified me. I learned that people some people die from the flu. I've been monitoring my temperature throughout the day. I might have a fever but I can't be sure. My throat feels scratchy. I'm too scared to get a flu shot because I heard it can make you sick. I live alone but I've been wearing a protective facemask and gloves around the apartment, just to be on the safe side. I wash my hands a lot with hand sanitizer. I'm afraid to go out. With all this talk of flu, I'm getting too scared to ride the bus to work because there are germs everywhere from people coughing into their hands and then touching things.

Health anxiety refers to the tendency to become alarmed by illness-related stimuli, including but not limited to, illness related to infectious diseases (Abramowitz & Braddock, 2011; Taylor & Asmundson, 2004). Health anxiety ranges on a continuum from mild to severe, and can be a state or a trait. The latter is a relatively enduring tendency. Our focus is on trait health anxiety.

Some people have very low levels of health anxiety. Their lack of concern about health risks can be maladaptive (e.g., neglecting to take necessary health precautions). Excessively low health concerns can be associated with an unrealistic optimism bias, as discussed in the previous chapter. People who are unconcerned about infection tend to neglect to perform recommended hygienic behaviors, such as washing their hands after using the washroom (Gilles et al., 2011) and tend to be nonadherent to social distancing (Goodwin, Gaines, Myers, & Neto, 2009; Jones & Salathe, 2009; Rubin et al., 2009; Williams, Rasmussen, Kleczkowski, Maharaj, & Cairns, 2015; Wong & Sam, 2011).

Excessively high health anxiety is characterized by undue anxiety or worry about one's health. That is, a disproportionate concern, given one's objective level of health. People with excessively high levels of health anxiety, compared to less anxious people, tend to become unduly alarmed by all kinds of perceived health threats, and overestimate the likelihood and seriousness of becoming ill (Hedman et al., 2016; Taylor & Asmundson, 2004; Wheaton, Berman, Franklin, & Abramowitz, 2010). Excessive health anxiety is associated with high levels of functional impairment and high levels of healthcare service utilization, even after controlling for physical comorbidities (Bobevski, Clarke, & Meadows, 2016; Eilenberg, Frostholm, Schroder, Jensen, & Fink, 2015; Sunderland, Newby, & Andrews, 2013). Vulnerability factors discussed in the previous chapter can contribute to the development of excessive health anxiety.

Excessive health anxiety—as seen in psychiatric disorders such as hypochondriasis, illness anxiety disorder, and somatic symptom disorder (American Psychiatric Association, 2000, 2013)—is common, with an estimated lifetime prevalence of 6% in the community (Sunderland et al., 2013). People prone to excessive health anxiety are likely to become particularly anxious during a threatened or actual epidemic or pandemic, as illustrated by the vignette at the beginning of this chapter. Such people may misinterpret somatic stress reactions (e.g., sweating, hot flushes, increased muscle tension) as signs of infection. The vignette also illustrates the nocebo effect, which occurs when negative expectations about treatment (e.g., a vaccination injection) cause the patient to experience negative side effects (Data-Franco & Berk, 2013; Kennedy, 1961; Petrie, Moss-Morris, Grey, & Shaw, 2004). Traits such as negative emotionality (neuroticism) may predispose people to experience the nocebo effect (Data-Franco & Berk, 2013).

Cognitive-behavioral models of health anxiety were developed in order to better understand various issues concerning healthcare utilization and medically unexplained physical symptoms (Leventhal,

Phillips, & Burns, 2016; Salkovskis & Warwick, 2001; Taylor & Asmundson, 2017). These models are also relevant to understanding other emotional reactions to pandemics. Such models propose that several cognitive and behavioral factors play a role in shaping the severity of health anxiety: Misinterpretations of health-related stimuli, maladaptive or distorted beliefs, memory and attention processes, and maladaptive behaviors.

Misinterpretations of Health-related Stimuli

Cognitive-behavioral models propose that excessive anxiety about one's health is triggered by the misinterpretation of health-related stimuli. Such stimuli include (1) bodily changes or sensations, which may or may not be indications of disease (e.g., fatigue, muscle aches), (2) direct health-related observations of other people (e.g., observing other people coughing or sneezing, or observing others becoming alarmed about being ill), and (3) more abstract forms of health-related information, such as warnings from one's doctor, advice from friends or family members, and information from social and mass media (e.g., newspaper reports about particular diseases).

Misinterpretations of the meaning of bodily changes or sensations include appraisals about the causes, time-course, seriousness, and control of the sensations (e.g., "My aching muscles mean that I'm getting the flu"). Evidence indicates that such appraisals influence a person's emotional reactions (e.g., anxiety, fear) and behavioral reactions (e.g., coping responses such as seeking out medical care) (Gautreau et al., 2015; Hagger, Koch, Chatzisarantis, & Orbell, 2017). People with excessive health anxiety tend to misinterpret harmless bodily sensations as dangerous. They may misinterpret bodily changes or sensations as signs of influenza, depending on their previous experiences with influenza and the information they have about any current strain of infection. Highly publicized disease outbreaks can lead medically healthy individuals, especially those with high levels of health anxiety, to misinterpret benign bodily changes and sensations (e.g., misinterpreting benign fatigue) as indicating that they have become infected, causing them to become unduly anxious (Taylor & Asmundson, 2004; Wheaton et al., 2012).

Beliefs about Health and Disease

Interpretations of health-related stimuli are influenced by memory processes such as recollections of past experiences (e.g., "My muscle aches in the past almost always meant I was getting sick") and by longstanding beliefs (e.g., beliefs such as "Chest tightness is always a sign of serious illness") (Salkovskis & Warwick, 2001; Taylor & Asmundson, 2004). Learning experiences (e.g., experiences of being hospitalized as a child) can lead some people to mistakenly believe that their health is fragile (Taylor & Asmundson, 2004).

People with excessive health anxiety tend to believe that all bodily sensations or bodily changes are potential signs of disease (Taylor & Asmundson, 2004). In the case of influenza, grossly inaccurate beliefs can contribute to excessive health anxiety. Such beliefs are unfortunately commonplace. To illustrate, in a survey of American college students conducted in the early stages of the 2009 Swine flu pandemic (Kanadiya & Sallar, 2011), 25% wrongly believed that Swine flu could be transmitted via water sources, 18% wrongly believed that Swine flu could be spread by insect bites, and 9% wrongly believed that Swine flu could be transmitted by eating cooked pork.

Focus of Attention

Attentional processes are important cognitive factors in shaping the intensity of health anxiety (Norris & Marcus, 2014; Witthöft et al., 2016). People with excessive health anxiety tend to be hypervigilant to bodily changes and sensations; that is, they pay a lot of attention to their bodies and therefore are likely to notice benign bodily perturbations (Tyrer & Tyrer, 2018). Consider, for example, a person who focuses attention on her breathing because she believes she might have a chest infection. This selective attention increases the odds of noticing bodily changes or sensations. During the 2014-2015 Ebola outbreak in West Africa, the fear of infection led people to persistently focus on their bodies, leading many people to misinterpret benign bodily changes or sensations as the first symptoms of Ebola virus disease (Desclaux et al., 2017).

Selective attention to bodily states is influenced not only by internal factors (i.e., sensations, beliefs, expectations), but also by external stimuli. People are more likely to detect bodily sensations if they are in environments in which there are few or no distractions (e.g., a windowless, undecorated hospital waiting room), as compared to an environment with numerous stimuli that attract the person's attention (e.g., a clinic waiting area with a window, wall hangings, and television) (Taylor & Asmundson, 2004).

Adaptive and Maladaptive Coping

People's interpretations influence whether or not they seek treatment, and whether they seek *appropriate* treatment. People can hold erroneous beliefs about what is an effective treatment. Some people believe that they only need symptomatic relief (e.g., cough suppressant medications), which may be insufficient if the underlying disease needs to be treated (Leventhal et al., 2016). People's appraisals of risk are often inaccurate. Indeed, there is only a weak correlation between people's anxiety about a particular risk and objective probability of death or harm (Frost, Frank, & Maibach, 1997; Young, Norman, & Humphreys, 2008).

People with high levels of health anxiety sometimes regard clinics as a source of sickness rather than a resource for help. This is illustrated in the following verbatim account provided by one health-anxious person:

> I'm afraid to go to the clinic, like if you are sick, like if you have colds, you would avoid going to see the doctors, because who knows, somebody before you has seen the doctors and left something, and then you go to see the doctors and you might [get] SARS. (Lee, 2014, p. 130)

People with excessive anxiety about infection tend to engage in maladaptive safety behaviors (i.e., behaviors intended to keep themselves safe) such as excessive hand washing and repeatedly seeking reassurance from medical professionals (Wheaton et al., 2012). Excessive handwashing can impair functioning in other areas of life (e.g., occupational functioning), especially when people devote hours per day to unnecessary handwashing. Excessive reassurance-seeking (e.g., repeatedly and unnecessarily seeking assurances that one is not sick) can add an unnecessary burden on the healthcare system. Excessive reassurance-seeking also can perpetuate health anxiety because (1) it increases the risk that the person will obtain conflicting medical information, (2) increases the risk of iatrogenic interventions, and (3) reinforces the person's view that their health is at risk (Salkovskis & Warwick, 2001; Taylor & Asmundson, 2004). The latter can occur, for example, when unnecessary medical tests (e.g., laboratory tests) are given in an attempt to reassure the anxious patient. The testing can be misinterpreted by the patient (e.g., "My doctor wouldn't be doing all these tests if she didn't think something was wrong"). Reassurance-seeking can consist of persistent searching the Internet for medical information ("cyberchondria"; Mathes, Norr, Allan, Albanese, & Schmidt, 2018), which increases the odds that the person will be exposed to alarming, false information (Taylor & Asmundson, 2004). People with excessive health anxiety also tend to engage in "doctor shopping"; that is, seeking consultations with multiple physicians so as to reassure themselves that they are not suffering from a serious disease. Doctor shopping places an undue burden on the medical system and increases the chances that the patient will receive seemingly conflicting or confusing medical advice (Taylor & Asmundson, 2004).

Treating Health Anxiety

Cognitive-behavioral models suggest that excessive health anxiety can be addressed by targeting dysfunctional beliefs and maladaptive behaviors. Consistent with this, randomized, controlled trials have shown that CBT is beneficial for people who suffer from excessive health anxiety (Cooper, Gregory, Walker, Lambe, & Salkovskis, 2017; Taylor, Asmundson, & Coons, 2005). Details of how to treat health anxiety with CBT are described elsewhere (e.g., Taylor & Asmundson, 2004). Other therapies have been used to treat excessive health anxiety, such as particular medications (e.g., selective serotonin reuptake inhibitors). However, such treatments have not been extensively evaluated in controlled studies. Bibliotherapy is another promising and sometimes useful intervention that requires further evaluation in randomized controlled trials (Tyrer & Tyrer, 2018). Here, CBT is present in booklet form, including information about the nature of health anxiety and various types of written and other exercises that the person can do to reduce his or her health anxiety (see, for example, Asmundson & Taylor, 2005). CBT, as conducted by a therapist, is currently the first-line treatment for excessive health anxiety (Taylor & Asmundson, 2017; Tyrer & Tyrer, 2018).

Conclusion

Health anxiety, defined as an enduring tendency or trait, varies on a continuum. Some people tend to have very low health anxiety, and therefore may fail to engage in basic hygiene or other recommended health measures (e.g., handwashing) because they do not perceive their health to be at risk. During times of pandemic, these people are liable to spread infection unless they can be persuaded to adhere to the health guidelines described in Chapter 2.

At the other end of the continuum, some people tend to have recurrent episodes of excessive health anxiety, despite being physically healthy. Such people are likely to become highly anxious during a pandemic and are likely to engage in maladaptive behaviors such as excessive avoidance (e.g., remaining, unnecessarily, secluded at home, away from perceived sources of contagion) and are likely to engage in persistent, repetitive, and unnecessary seeking of medical reassurance. During a pandemic, this would place an added burden on an already over-taxed healthcare system. Excessive health anxiety can be effectively treated with CBT.

Chapter 6

The Behavioral Immune System

Detection and Avoidance of Sickly Others

Complementing the cognitive-behavioral approach to health anxiety, which focuses largely on dysfunctional beliefs and their effects, the concept of the behavioral immune system (BIS) focuses on basic motivational aspects of disease avoidance, whereby emotional states such as disgust are important motivators. The concept of the BIS further complements cognitive-behavioral models in that the BIS provides important insights into the social consequences of disease avoidance mechanisms.

Infectious agents such as bacteria and viruses are too small to be directly observed. Accordingly, a person's biological immune system is insufficient for avoiding exposure to pathogens. It is necessary to use perceptible cues to detect the presence of potentially harmful agents. Such cues include noxious smells and visual cues like the presence of people coughing or sneezing. The BIS is conceptualized as a system for detecting and reacting to such cues. The BIS is a complex suite of cognitive, affective, and behavioral mechanisms that help prevent pathogen transmission in the face of recurrent infectious disease threats (Ackerman, Hill, & Murray, 2018; Schaller & Park, 2011). The BIS consists of conscious and non-conscious psychological mechanisms that detect cues to the presence of infectious pathogens in the immediate environment, and trigger disease-relevant emotional responses (e.g., fear, disgust) and other responses that motivate disease avoidance (Schaller & Park, 2011).

The BIS is said to have evolved to minimize potentially fatal failures to detect pathogens. Such failures are minimized if the system is biased towards false positives (false alarms) in detecting pathogens. This is similar to an overly sensitive biological immune system that triggers an immune response to harmless agents (e.g., allergic reactions triggered by dust or pollen). Thus, the BIS is sensitive to cues that only superficially resemble environmental signs of infection. The BIS is proposed to be especially sensitive when people perceive themselves to be vulnerable to infection. Here, the person becomes especially attentive to cues that indicate that pathogens may be present, and these cues trigger responses such as disgust, fear, and the urge to escape (Schaller & Park, 2011).

Perceived Vulnerability to Disease

There are individual differences in BIS sensitivity (Duncan & Schaller, 2009; Duncan et al., 2009), as indicated by research on two correlated traits, which are markers of BIS sensitivity: Perceived vulnerability to disease (PVD) and disgust sensitivity. PVD refers to an individual's sense of personal vulnerability to infectious disease. Perceived vulnerability may be accurate or inaccurate, as compared to objective measures of the person's immunocompetence. When considering a person's emotional and behavioral reactions to the threat of pandemic infection, it is not so much the objective risk that is important but rather the person's perceived vulnerability to disease, because perceptions of threat determine the person's emotional and behavioral responses.

PVD is assessed by the Perceived Vulnerability to Disease Scale (PVDS), which consists of two correlated dimensions (subscales): (1) Perceived vulnerability to infectious disease (perceived infectability), and (2) avoidance and discomfort in situations in which a person is liable to be infected (germ aversion) (Duncan et al., 2009). The PVDS is a short (15-item) questionnaire that has performed well on tests of reliability and validity. As such, it is a promising means of identifying people at risk for adverse emotional reactions in response to the threat of pandemic infection. The dimensions of PVD, as measured by the PVDS, are uncorrelated with age, gender, or education, but are significantly correlated with various indices of psychopathology (e.g., negative emotionality) and with the tendency to worry about one's general health (e.g., Clay, 2017; Diaz, Soriano, & Belena, 2016; Duncan et al., 2009; Magallares, Fuster-Ruiz De Apodaca, & Morales, 2017). During the 2005 Avian flu outbreak, scores on the PVDS germ aversion scale predicted fears of contracting Avian flu (Green et al., 2010). Overall, the findings suggest that people with high levels of PVD are at risk of becoming highly distressed during a pandemic.

Disgust Sensitivity

Another marker of BIS sensitivity is disgust sensitivity, which is the degree of emotional distress and revulsion a person tends to experience when confronted with disgust-evoking stimuli, such as stimuli related to disease, contamination, or the bodily products of other people or animals (e.g., mucus, saliva, or fecal matter; Goetz, Lee, Cougle, & Turkel, 2013). Research suggests that there is a universal set of disgust cues. These include bodily wastes, body contents, sick, deformed, dead or unhygienic people, some sexual behaviors, dirty environments, certain foods—especially if spoiled or unfamiliar—and particular animals (Curtis, de Barra, & Aunger, 2011). Objects that have contacted any of the above can also be experienced as disgusting. People are disgusted not only by things that pose a real risk of pathogen infection (e.g., dog feces), they also are disgusted by things that pose no risk at all but that simply bear some superficial resemblance to real risks (e.g., chocolate fudge sculpted into the shape of dog feces; Oaten, 2009; Rozin, Haidt, & McCauley, 2008).

Disgust sensitivity varies between individuals as a trait and within individuals as a state (Curtis et al., 2011). Here, we focus on disgust sensitivity as a trait. Research conducted during the 2009 Swine flu pandemic found that disgust sensitivity predicted a person's fear of acquiring influenza (Brand, McKay, Wheaton, & Abramowitz, 2013; Wheaton et al., 2012). Disgust sensitivity is also correlated with contamination-related obsessive-compulsive disorder and with various phobias, including phobias of blood, injury, or injections (Ludvik, Boschen, & Neumann, 2015; Olatunji, Cisler, McKay, & Phillips, 2010). This suggests that some people who become highly anxious during a pandemic—that is, those people with elevated disgust sensitivity—are also likely to have other, preexisting types of anxiety-related psychopathology.

Pathogens and Prejudice

A common way of contracting infection is from other humans, especially when foreign groups intermingle, in which one group introduces a disease which the other group has never encountered and has no immunity against (Navarrete & Fessler, 2006). European explorers to the Americas, for example, brought smallpox, influenza, and other viruses, which decimated the indigenous inhabitants

(Pringle, 2015). Given that many infections are transmitted through interpersonal interactions, the BIS is said to have evolved to influence social attitudes and interactions, including ethnocentrism and negative attitudes toward immigrants and other foreigners (Schaller & Park, 2011). Consistent with this, many studies have shown that when people feel threatened about becoming infected with some pathogen, they tend to avoid or stigmatize out-groups (i.e., groups which a person does not belong to, or identify with) (Ackerman et al., 2018; Faulkner, Schaller, Park, & Duncan, 2004; Joffe, 1999; Makhanova, Miller, & Maner, 2015). Thus, out-groups are blamed for causing or spreading diseases, such as being blamed for lack of hygiene, education, self-control, or other factors such as cultural practices (Gilles et al., 2013). Moreover, people who feel especially vulnerable to infection—that is, people who perceive themselves as highly vulnerable to disease (i.e., high scores on the PVDS)—are most likely to avoid foreigners and have negative attitudes toward such people (Aarøe, Petersen, & Arceneaux, 2017; Duncan, Schaller, & Park, 2009; Faulkner et al., 2004; Green et al., 2010; Navarrete & Fessler, 2006; Schaller & Park, 2011). Perceived threat of infection is also associated with prejudice toward people who display superficial characteristics correlated with poor health, such as a physical disability, obesity, and old age (Duncan & Schaller, 2009; Park, Faulkner, & Schaller, 2003; Park, Schaller, & Crandall, 2007; White, Johnson, & Kwan, 2014).

If a population is threatened with severe infection, the BIS will be activated in almost everyone, with some people having particularly intense levels of activation. This suggests that during times of pandemic there will be a general increase in stigmatization and xenophobia, where foreigners and other out-groups are blamed for being sources of infection (Murray & Schaller, 2012). Indeed, this was observed during the SARS epidemic, in which the British media erroneously attributed SARS to unhygienic Chinese cultural habits, such as dirty markets, living in close proximity to animals, and the habit of spitting on the ground (Washer, 2004). Similarly, stigmatization occurred during the Bubonic Plague in Italy. In 1576 in Milan, for example, the homes of Jews were subjected to health inspections because of prejudicial beliefs that these people were sources of contagion (Cohn, 2010).

Visible minorities are not the only people that may be stigmatized during outbreaks of infectious disease. HCWs who care for patients with serious infectious diseases are commonly stigmatized because of their disease exposure. To illustrate, about 20% of HCWs involved in the SARS outbreak in Taiwan reported feeling stigmatized and rejected by their neighbors (Bai et al., 2004). During the SARS outbreak in Singapore, 49% of HCWs experienced stigmatization because of their jobs (Koh et al., 2005). Even survivors of SARS were stigmatized; for example, shunned by co-workers, even though they had fully recovered (Cheng, 2004).

Infection-related prejudice against out-groups can be associated with the belief in conspiracy theories (see Chapter 7) about the role of foreigners or healthcare authorities in the spreading of disease (Atlani-Duault, Mercier, Rousseau, Guyot, & Moatti, 2015). The Ebola conspiratorial beliefs in West Africa were discussed in Chapter 1, where rumors spread that foreigners (HCWs and journalists) were deliberately harming patients in treatment facilities (Quick, 2018). An analogous situation arose in 2010 in Haiti, during an unexpected outbreak of cholera, the first in many decades. Some Haitians believed that the disease was deliberately spread by foreigners and other malevolent agents (Grimaud & Legagneur, 2011).

Disease-related stigma is important for many obvious reasons. Stigma is a mark of social disgrace (Goffman, 1963). During outbreaks of serious infectious disease, stigma against particular groups (e.g., visible minorities) can have several effects: (1) Stigma is stressful and distressing; (2) it creates barriers to healthcare (e.g., concerns about discrimination from healthcare providers may dissuade people from seeking care); (3) stigma can lead to social marginalization, which can lead to poverty and neglect, thereby reducing early detection and treatment and furthering the spread of disease; (4) stigmatized people may distrust health authorities and resist cooperation during a public health emergency; and (5) stigma may distort public perceptions of risk, resulting in undue anxiety, avoidance, and economic costs (e.g., fear and avoidance of Asian stores and Asian areas of town during the SARS outbreak, as discussed above) (Barrett & Brown, 2008; Crocker, Major, & Steele, 1998; Schibalski et al., 2017).

Implications for Naming Diseases

The concept of the BIS has important implications for the naming of diseases. Terms such as "Swine flu" and "Asian flu" have become standard labels for pandemics. However, such labels should be used with caution because of the important psychological implications of naming pandemics after animals, geographic regions, or nationalities. Such naming conventions can lead to misconceptions among the public and can amplify discrimination and stigmatization during times of pandemic.

Conclusion

The concept of the BIS is useful for understanding emotional and motivational reactions when people perceive themselves to be threatened with infection. The BIS is particularly useful in understanding societal reactions to the threat of infection, particularly discrimination against out-groups (e.g., foreigners) and people who appear to be in poor health or appear to have been somehow associated with an infectious agent. As predicted by the concept of the BIS, when threatened with infection, people may react with xenophobia and may stigmatize particular groups. Stigma and discrimination can be an added source of distress to people struggling to cope with pandemic infection.

CBT can reduce PVD (Taylor & Asmundson, 2004), and can reduce associated features such as disgust sensitivity (Ludvik et al., 2015; Olatunji & McKay, 2009). CBT might also reduce the downstream effects of PVD such as the tendency to discriminate against out-groups. If this is the case then CBT would be doubly important during the next pandemic for reducing both health anxiety and discrimination. CBT would not be sufficient on a community-wide scale, however, because there would not be sufficient resources to deliver this therapy on such a wide scale. Future research is needed to determine how the findings concerning the BIS and PVD can be translated into community programs for reducing discrimination.

CHAPTER 7

CONSPIRACY THEORIES

What are Conspiracy Theories?

> To think of all conspiracy theorists as cranks is not helpful—there are just too many (Weigmann, 2018, p. 2).

During the next pandemic, we can expect to see the emergence of various conspiracy theories about the source or cause of the infectious agent and about the vaccines (if available) used to treat it. As for conspiracy theories in general, they are attempts to explain the causes of significant events by claiming they are due to secret plots by powerful actors (Douglas, Sutton, & Cichocka, 2017). Conspiracy beliefs refer to beliefs in a specific conspiracy theory or set of theories. The belief in conspiracy theories is remarkably widespread. About 60% of Americans believe President John F. Kennedy was killed in a conspiracy involving the Mafia, CIA, or the government (Swift, 2013). More than a third of Americans believe in the conspiracy theory that climate change is a hoax, perpetrated by vested interest groups such as climate scientists in need of research funding (Douglas et al., 2019). Belief in conspiracy theories appears to be a culturally universal phenomenon (van Prooijen & van Vugt, 2018).

Medical Conspiracy Theories

Disease outbreaks are commonly the subject of conspiracy theories, especially when the nature of the disease is poorly understood. Regarding the AIDS pandemic, for example, there have been several unsubstantiated conspiracy theories contending that HIV/AIDS is a bioengineered weapon intended to wipe out homosexuality or to commit racial genocide by eliminating African Americans (Heller, 2015; Parsons, Simmons, Shinhoster, & Kilburn, 1999). In Padua, Italy, during the Bubonic Plague outbreak of 1576, a pamphlet was circulated widely in the city, proclaiming the conspiracy theory that "wicked ones (*sciagurati*) were spreading the disease intentionally with infected clothing and poisonous ointments (*untioni*) rubbed on door handles and knockers" (Cohn, 2010, p. 119). During the Spanish flu pandemic, which occurred during World War I, there was a conspiracy theory that the virus was being spread by a pharmaceutical company:

> Such was the virulence of anti-German fanaticism in 1918 that the USPHS [United States Public Health Service] was obliged ... to test Bayer Aspirin tablets to counteract rumors that Bayer, producing aspirin under what had originally been a German patent, was poisoning its customers with flu germs. The tablets proved to be uninhabited [by germs]. (Crosby, 2003, p. 216)

Conspiracy theories were also raised about the Zika virus. According to one unsubstantiated theory, the virus was the inadvertent creation of a biotech company that had been raising genetically modified mosquitoes to combat dengue fever (Jacobs, Perpetua, Sreeharsha, McNeil, & Tavernise, 2016). Another unsubstantiated theory asserted that Zika was part of a plot by global elites—a shadowy organization known as the New World Order—to depopulate the planet and install a one-world government (Jacobs et al., 2016). There is no evidence that this organization ever existed but it has, nonetheless, been the focus of numerous conspiracy theories. According to one theory, the New World Order was responsible for the SARS outbreak (Lee, 2014). Early in the SARS outbreak, Australian health officials were forced to quell conspiracy theories about SARS being an act of terrorism or biological warfare conducted by some malevolent country or agency (Lee, 2014). During the 2009 Swine flu pandemic various conspiracy theories arose, including the theory that terrorists were using infected Mexicans immigrating to the United States as "walking germ warfare weapons" (Smallman, 2015, p. 5).

A survey of a nationally representative sample of 1,351 American adults revealed that a sizable minority of people believe in medically unsubstantiated conspiracy theories (Oliver & Wood, 2014), as indicated by the proportion of US adults agreeing with the following conspiracy theories:

- The Food and Drug Administration is deliberately preventing the public from getting natural cures for cancer and other diseases because of pressure from drug companies: 37% agreed.

- Health officials know that cell phones cause cancer but are doing nothing to stop it because large corporations won't let them: 20% agreed.
- The global dissemination of genetically modified foods by the Monsanto corporation is part of a secret program, called Agenda 21, launched by the Rockefeller and Ford foundations to shrink the world's population: 12% agreed.
- Public water fluoridation is really just a secret way for chemical companies to dump dangerous byproducts of phosphate mines into the environment: 12% agreed.
- Doctors and the government still want to vaccinate children even though they know these vaccines cause autism and other psychological disorders: 20% agreed.

Causes and Correlates of Conspiratorial Thinking

Conspiracy theories are most likely to arise during times of uncertainty about important events, especially if the events are threatening and personally relevant (Wood, 2018). Conspiracy theories typically emerge in marked opposition to particular mainstream or official accounts. Such theories can provide a simple, understandable picture of a personally relevant threatening, uncertain situation: Why something happened, who benefits from it, and who should be blamed (Weigmann, 2018; Wood, 2018). Conspiracy theories are resistant to falsification in that they postulate that conspirators use stealth and disinformation to cover up their actions, which implies that people who try to debunk conspiracy theories may, themselves, be part of the conspiracy (Douglas et al., 2017).

People differ not only in the degree to which they believe in specific conspiracy theories, but also in their susceptibility to such theories in general (Bruder, Haffke, Neave, Nouripanah, & Imhoff, 2013). People who believe in one conspiracy theory tend to believe in others (Douglas et al., 2019; Galliford & Furnham, 2017; Lewandowsky, Oberauer, & Gignac, 2013). For example, people who believe that the Zika virus is spread by Monsanto also tend to believe that 9/11 was an inside job, that NASA faked the moon landings, and that governments are covering up evidence of extraterrestrial contact.

Conspiracy theories, as promulgated on social media (e.g., Twitter, Facebook, YouTube) and through other avenues, have several common features: (1) The proponents typically go to great efforts to cite supposedly authoritative sources to support their claims, even if such claims might be vague (e.g., "Research at Harvard has shown that…"); (2) the theories themselves are often vague; and (3) the proponents frequently use leading questions; a "just asking" style in which they raise rhetorical questions to challenge mainstream views (e.g., "If vaccines are so safe, then how do you explain the increase in disease X in country when people received the vaccine Z?") (Wood, 2018).

Evidence suggests that the tendency to believe in conspiracy theories is driven by motives that can be characterized as *epistemic* (needing to understand one's environment), *existential* (needing to feel safe and in control of one's environment), and *social* (needing to maintain a positive image of oneself and one's in-group) (Douglas et al., 2017). Conspiracy theories tend to be particularly appealing to people who find the positive image of their self or in-group to be threatened (Cichocka, Marchlewska, Golec de Zavala, & Olechowski, 2016; Douglas et al., 2017).

A large number of studies have investigated the individual difference variables that predict a person's tendency to believe in conspiracy theories (e.g., Bruder et al., 2013; Cichocka, Marchlewska, & Golec de Zavala, 2016; Craft, Ashley, & Maksl, 2017; Douglas et al., 2017, 2019; Galliford & Furnham, 2017; Imhoff & Lamberty, 2018; Lahrach & Furnham, 2017; Lantian, Muller, Nurra, & Douglas, 2017; Marchlewska, Cichocka, & Kossowska, 2018; Moulding et al., 2016; Swami, Voracek, Stieger, Tran, & Furnham, 2014). Research shows that the tendency to believe in conspiracy theories is correlated with the following:

- Suspiciousness, magical thinking, and the tendency to believe in the paranormal.
- Narcissism (i.e., an inflated view of oneself that requires external validation) and the need to feel unique that can be fulfilled by believing that one has special knowledge about conspiracies.
- Worry about one's health and mortality, for people who believe in medical conspiracy theories.
- Gullibility, lower media literacy (i.e., poorer ability to critically analyze the source and contents of news stories, as indicated, for example, by the tendency to believe in fake news), lower intelligence, lower education, and poorer skills in analytical thinking.

- Rejection of conventional scientific findings or theories (e.g., the theory of evolution) in favor of pseudoscience (e.g., the belief that prayer is effective in curing terminal disease).

Overall, the research suggests that conspiracy theories appeal to people who seek accuracy or meaning about personally important issues, but lack the cognitive resources or have other problems that prevent them from finding the answers to questions by more rational means (Douglas et al., 2019). Conspiracy theories may also allow people to feel that they possess rare, important information that other people do not have, making them feel special and thus boosting their self-esteem.

Methods for Reducing Conspiratorial Thinking

In some cases, it may be very difficult, if not impossible to persuade people to abandon their conspiratorial beliefs, such as beliefs about the causes of a given virus. However, research suggests that people can be inoculated against conspiracy theories by being exposed to arguments that refute conspiracy theories, before the person is exposed to pro-conspiracy arguments (Jolley & Douglas, 2017). Techniques that stimulate analytical thinking also can reduce the belief in conspiracies (Swami et al., 2014). But once the belief in a conspiracy theory is firmly established, it can be difficult to correct (Jolley & Douglas, 2017). Motivational interviewing and related approaches such as motivational enhancement therapy can be used to target conspiratorial thinking (Hornsey & Fielding, 2017; Miller & Rollnick, 2013). These methods are applied on an individual basis, such as during therapy. It is unclear how they could be applied on a community-wide basis.

Conclusion

Conspiracy theories arise during times of uncertainty in order for people make sense of threatening events. People differ in their tendency to embrace conspiracy theories and there are various reasons why people engage in conspiratorial thinking. Medical conspiracy theories may lead to vaccine nonadherence and may fuel pandemic-related anxiety. Therefore, conspiracy theories would be important to address in the next pandemic. However, a person need not believe in conspiracy theories in order to be anxious during a pandemic. Their anxiety might be realistic or might arise from an exaggerated estimate of the degree of threat, without engaging in conspiratorial thinking. For such pandemic-related distress, emotional vulnerability factors may be more important, including trait anxiety and intolerance of uncertainty. These traits are not consistently related to the belief in conspiracy theories (Grzesiak-Feldman, 2013; Moulding et al., 2016; Swami et al., 2014) but predict who will become distressed when threatened with infection, such as pandemic influenza. So, although conspiratorial thinking is an important issue, there are other issues of equal and perhaps greater importance.

CHAPTER 8

SOCIAL PSYCHOLOGICAL FACTORS

How do Beliefs and Fears Spread Through Social Networks?

Beliefs and fears about diseases, just like diseases themselves, spread through social networks. Beliefs also influence the spread of infection. If there is widespread belief in the importance of handwashing, for example, then this will curtail the spread of disease. In general, beliefs and fears are spread in three main ways: (1) Information transmission, such as by media reports (e.g., text, images) or verbal information received from other people (e.g., rumors); (2) direct personal experiences, including conditioning events (e.g., exposure to trauma); and (3) observational learning (e.g., witnessing other people acting frightened in response to some stimulus) (Barlow, 2004; Goumon & Špinka, 2016). Information transmission and observational learning are particularly relevant to the spread of beliefs and fears through social networks.

Rumors

A rumor, as the term is defined in the social sciences, refers to a "story or piece of information of unknown reliability that is passed from person to person" (Vandenbos, 2007, p. 808). Rumors are "improvised news" (Shibutani, 1966), spreading rapidly when the demand for information exceeds the supply, as is the case during times of uncertainty about important issues. Rumors may be spread if they help people make sense of an ambiguous situation, such as the possible threat of infection, and if rumors offer guidance about how to cope with the perceived risks (DiFonzo & Bordia, 2007; Rosnow, Esposito, & Gibney, 1988).

Rumors can arise from anonymous sources, causing uncertainty about the veracity of the information. Traditionally, rumors were spread by word-of-mouth but now are spread by the mass media and social media. Rumors, as they pass with retelling, tend to become shorter and simpler (e.g., details are omitted), sharpened (e.g., some details are accentuated or exaggerated), and altered in a way that matches cultural stereotypes, expectations and biases (Allport & Postman, 1947; DiFonzo & Bordia, 2007). Rumors and their management are issues of practical importance because unchecked rumors can lead, for example, to widespread fear, hostility and suspicion, and social disruption.

Rumors may be true, false, or somewhere in between. Some rumors may involve urban myths or stories that might seem highly plausible. An urban myth is illustrated in the following incident, which occurred during the 1918 Spanish flu pandemic, which occurred during World War I.

> In the context of the raging war in Europe, residents of Baltimore like many Americans expressed their anti-German sentiments by characterizing the disease as an immoral, murderous "Hun of a disease" and by entertaining rumors that German spies were infiltrating the country and spreading the sickness. The local incarnation of this rumor took the form of a "nurse of German extraction" who was caught distributing germs in the hospital wards of Camp Meade and later executed. (Schoch-Spana, 2004, p. 47)

There was no documented evidence of any such nurse. During the same pandemic in England, *The Times* erroneously reported a rumor that the Spanish flu was "directly traceable to the German use of poison gas, the after-effects of which have induced the growth of a new type of streptococcus" (Johnson, 2006, p. 186). Again, there was no evidence to support this rumor.

A similarly false rumor was spread about the prevalence of SARS in New York City's Chinatown (Eichelberger, 2007). Even without a single case of SARS in Chinatown, the area was quickly identified as a hotspot of contagion and risk. "The American public, including Chinatown, had become infected with an epidemic of fear, not of disease" (Eichelberger, 2007, p. 1285).

Rumors can be spread maliciously and to promote prejudice. During the 2003 SARS epidemic, for example, a hoaxer in Hong Kong posted a bogus news item on a faux news site, claiming that Hong Kong would soon be declared an infected region and sealed off from the rest of the world. Such a rumor quickly spread around the city, causing frightened people to rush to stores to purchase supplies (Cheng & Cheung, 2005).

Note that there are many similarities between rumors and conspiracy theories. In some ways, a conspiracy theory is an extreme, highly specific form of rumor. Methods for managing rumors are discussed in Chapter 9.

Observational Learning

Emotional contagion, including the spread of fear, is a basic building block of human interaction, allowing people to understand and share the feelings of others by "feeling themselves into" another person's emotions (Hatfield, Carpenter, & Rapson, 2014). Research shows that observational learning is an important way in which emotions, including fears, are spread (Bandura, 1986; Debiec & Olsson, 2017). Observational learning involves the acquisition of information, skills, or behavior by watching the performance of others. Fears may be acquired via observational learning, such as by seeing or hearing people express fear about some issue, such as a possible pandemic. Observational learning can include seeing fearful faces or bodily postures and hearing frightened voices. Studies show that exposure to social cues signaling threat, such as the sight or sound of a scared person, can trigger or amplify fear, which is a phenomenon known as fear contagion (Debiec & Olsson, 2017). Research also shows that people can also "smell fear"; that is, people can detect olfactory fear cues given off by the sweat of frightened individuals. Experiments show that these olfactory cues can elicit fear in other people (de Groot, Semin, & Smeets, 2014).

The perception of a common threat can lead to behavioral mimicry of fear reactions, thereby promoting the spreading of fear (Gump & Kulik, 1997). This is not unique to fear. Research suggests that humans, being social animals, tend to spontaneously and automatically mimic the behavior of other people, including facial expressions, body movements, and vocal expressions (Hatfield et al., 2014). Afferent feedback from such facial or postural mimicry can induce, in an attenuated form, the corresponding emotions (e.g., behaving in a frightened way can induce the emotion of fear) (Hatfield, Cacioppo, & Rapson, 1994; Hatfield et al., 2014).

Evidence suggests that some combination of observational learning and information transmission plays a role in pandemic-related fear. Research conducted during the 2009 Swine flu pandemic, for example, showed that children's fear of Swine flu was predicted by their parent's fear of Swine flu (Remmerswaal & Muris, 2011). The parent's transmission of threat information was positively correlated with children's fear. This link remained significant even after controlling for other sources of information (i.e., from media, friends, and school) and direct experience with the disease.

News Media

News media outlets attempt to deal with a vast quantity of news information by filtering it into a few columns in the daily newspapers or into a few sound bites on the nightly news. News reports both reflect and reinforce community anxieties and concerns (Bird, 1996). The news media has been long accused of exaggerating dangers, thereby creating undue public fear (Kilgo et al., 2018). During the 2002-2003 SARS outbreak, for example, the media exaggerated the dangerousness and contagiousness of the virus, leading to widespread but short-lived public anxiety and xenophobia (Muzzatti, 2005).

> News coverage in the United States saturated viewers with images of East and Southeast Asians wearing masks and creatively-framed camera angles provided footage of deserted Chinatowns in American urban centers, further fueling the stigma. (Muzzatti 2005, p. 123)

Noticeably absent from most media coverage was the fact that SARS was not easily communicable, nor was it fatal in the majority of cases (Muzzatti, 2005). As a side note, the SARS outbreak was curiously self-limiting. The coronavirus causing SARS disappeared from the human population as abruptly as it had arrived, before a vaccine or cure could be found (Lee, 2014).

During the 2004-2007 outbreak of Avian flu, the news media was criticized for exaggerating the risk and lethality of infections by using emotionally toned language, making misleading comparisons between the Avian flu and the deadlier Spanish flu, the misuse (selective use) of statistics, along with questionable estimates of death toll and cost of infectious outbreaks (Abeysinghe & White, 2010).

When the 2009 Swine flu pandemic proved to be not as lethal as initially feared, some commentators blamed the media (and health officials) for exaggerating the threat (Bonneux & Van Damme, 2010; Keil, Schönhöfer, & Spelsberg, 2011). However, an analysis of media reports suggests a more nuanced interpretation. Klemm, Das, and Hartmann (2016) conducted a systematic review of previously published content-analytic studies of media reports concerning the Swine flu pandemic. Klemm et al. developed a coding scheme specifying three indicators of dramatized media coverage: (1) The *volume* of media coverage (i.e., extensive coverage may serve as risk amplifier, regardless of whether the risk is portrayed accurately), (2) the media *content* presented, particularly an overemphasis of threat while neglecting measures of self-protection, and (3) the *tone* of coverage. Tone refers to dramatic or sensational use of emotion-laden descriptions (e.g., discussion of worst-case scenarios of what "might" happen) and use of particular attention-grabbing production features such as special effects (e.g., sound effects, fast cutting of some scenes, slow-motion effects for others), which can exaggerate factual content (Klemm et al., 2016). Results indicated that media attention was immense, that news content stressed threat over precautionary measures, while there was inconsistent evidence for the use of an overly dramatic or sensational tone. This led Klemm and colleagues to conclude that the media may have contributed to heightened risk perceptions primarily through a high volume of coverage and an unbalanced emphasis on the threat of Swine flu.

Experts interviewed for the media can also add to the sensationalism in news reports. When commenting on the Avian flu outbreak, for example, a prominent British virologist was quoted in *The Guardian* as saying "Forget al-Qaeda, the biggest terrorist threat we face today is Mother Nature" (Nerlich & Halliday, 2007, p. 59). Thus, it is not possible to blame the media entirely for fueling fears about pandemics. Even so, the media may exaggerate the messages that experts or health authorities want to convey.

Complicating matters, exaggerated media reports lead to diverse reactions among the public. Some members of the public react with excessive fear, while others dismiss the new reports as gross exaggerations. Both types of reaction are common. To illustrate, a study of 1,027 Canadians found that, regarding the Swine flu pandemic, 45% believed that the media reports were reasonably accurate, 36% believed the reports were exaggerated, and the remaining 19% found the media reports to be contradictory or confusing (Taha et al., 2013). People who are skeptical of media reports are less likely to engage in health behaviors recommended by health authorities (Rubin et al., 2009).

Mass media fatigue can undermine efforts to curb the spread of infection (Collinson, Khan, & Heffernan, 2015). Although sensationalized news articles can promote anxiety, the pervasive media coverage of social problems can lead to desensitization; that is, a diminished emotional response to negative news reports (Collinson et al., 2015). People may follow the recommended health precautions during the initial phases of an outbreak but then become lax over time as they become desensitized to news reports. Little is known about the factors influencing mass media fatigue, beyond the finding that the sheer volume of exposure to news reports can influence mass media fatigue. There may be individual differences in proneness to such fatigue although this remains to be investigated.

It is unrealistic to expect reporters to avoid or remove all the journalistic devices used to sensationalize a news story. Responsible journalistic reporting is not devoid of reporting anxiety-inducing details. However, solutions, interventions, useful information for the public, and other anxiety-reducing elements are as important to cover as warnings and speculations. News reporters can reduce public fear by accentuating solutions and successful efforts to control and contain a health crisis (Kilgo et al., 2018).

Social Media

The use of social media—such as Facebook, Twitter, Reddit, and YouTube—is ubiquitous. Social media involve web and mobile-based technologies and platforms that enable the content creation, collaboration and sharing of information by members of the public. About two-thirds of US adults have a Facebook account, for example, and about half of those users obtain their news information from Facebook (Sharma, Yadav, Yadav, & Ferdinand, 2017). Social media have become a major source of health information for people worldwide and have become a global platform for outbreak and health risk communication (Adebayo, Neumark, Gesser-Edelsburg, Abu Ahmad, & Levine, 2017).

Traditional news services, such as newspapers and radio and television broadcasts, offer a one-way dissemination of information. Journalists and broadcasters simply deliver information to a receiving public. Social media have dramatically changed the way that news is spread. Social media users play an important gatekeeping role in information dissemination; users make decisions about what information to share and where to share it, may selectively share (amplify) some types of media coverage and ignore others, and may create their own content (Kilgo et al., 2018). Users who express interest in a particular news story, for example, by liking a post on Facebook, create social cues that signal the value of information to others (Strekalova, 2017). When sharing news articles, users who post to social media or social news sites can choose traditional media news or alternative (non-mainstream) news outlets. Thus, sharing provides the opportunity for user-generated content or alternative media sites to receive increased attention (Kilgo et al., 2018). Anyone can widely disseminate their opinion about almost anything.

Social media are a two-edged sword. They can rapidly disseminate information and misinformation. They can fuel or quell fears, and they can influence the spreading of disease by influencing people's behavior. This potentially raises problems with the spreading of excessive fear. The same can be said for modern communication technologies in general, including the Internet.

> When the next major pandemic strikes, it will be accompanied by something never before seen in human history: an explosion of billions of texts, tweets, e-mails, blogs, photos, and videos rocketing across the planet's computers and mobile devices. Some of these billions of words and pictures will have useful information, but many will be filled with rumors, innuendo, misinformation, and hyper-sensational claims. ... As a result, hundreds of millions of people will receive unvetted and incorrect assertions, uncensored images, and unqualified guidance, all of which, if acted on, could endanger their own health, seriously damage their economies, and undermine the stability of their societies. (Walker, 2016, p. 43)

A large volume of misleading information is posted on social media. Research indicates, for example, that about 20-30% of YouTube videos about emerging infectious diseases contain inaccurate or misleading information (Tang, Bie, Park, & Zhi, 2018). A survey of YouTube videos during the Zika virus pandemic found that 24% contained misleading information (Bora, Das, Barman, & Borah, 2018). An analysis of Facebook posts during the Zika pandemic further revealed that misleading posts were far more popular than posts presenting accurate, relevant public health information about the disease (Sharma et al., 2017). An analysis of Reddit posts during the 2014 Ebola outbreak in West Africa similarly revealed that news shared on Reddit was more sensational and tended to amplify anxiety and uncertainty, as compared to information presented in traditional newspaper coverage (Kilgo et al., 2018). Such findings are important because social media posts can influence people's emotions and behaviors.

How might social media be better used for health promotion during times of pandemic? Sharma et al. (2017) called for better curation of public health-related social media posts during times of health crises; that is, refraining from passing on sensational, speculative, or misleading information. But this would work only if the public voluntarily agreed not to circulate such news items. Imposed censorship of such material by moderators of social media sites would likely contribute to the spread of conspiracy theories. Sharma et al. (2017) suggested that misleading health information could be tagged (e.g., Facebook posts can be tagged) to indicate that it contains misleading, questionable, or unverified health information. Whether this would be feasible or successful remains to be seen.

Some researchers have recommended that health campaigns focus on recruiting influential Twitter accounts for retweeting accurate, health-promoting information (Yun et al., 2016). Tang et al. (2018) suggested enlisting alternative spokespersons such as celebrities. This seems problematic. The majority of media celebrities are not content experts and might just as easily pass on misleading information. There is also concern that the reliance on celebrities could undermine health literacy among some members of the general public. Health literacy refers to a person's knowledge, motivation, and competence to access, understand, critically appraise, and apply health information for their healthcare (Sørensen et al., 2012). People should be encouraged to seek out authoritative, reliable information sources rather than blindly accepting someone's advice simply because that person is some kind of celebrity.

Social Media and Vaccination Attitudes

Social media may contribute to the anti-vaccination movement by providing a vehicle for recruiting members and garnering media attention. Facebook anti-vaccination groups provide a form of "echo-chamber" where people can mutually support their anti-scientific views (Pilkington & Glenza, 2019). However, the relationship between social media and vaccination attitudes is more complex. Although the Internet makes it easy to spread and reinforce anti-vaccination beliefs and conspiracy theories, the Internet equally makes it easy to criticize such beliefs and theories. Conspiracy theory websites are not highly visited by the general public and have a far smaller audience than mainstream news sources (Douglas et al., 2019). There is some evidence, however, that some "vaccination skeptical" websites may be more effective in their methods of communication than pro-vaccination websites. One study, for example, compared two vaccination skeptical and two pro-vaccination websites and found that the former had links to both pro- and anti-vaccination information, creating the appearance that both sides of the issue were being presented openly (Grant et al., 2015). Unlike the pro-vaccination websites, the vaccination skeptical websites were highly interactive, providing a forum for community discussion. This suggests that the vaccination skeptical websites were more effective in fostering community building. Pro-vaccination websites provided limited interaction, focusing on imparting knowledge, which conspiracy theorists may view as aloof and dictatorial (Douglas et al., 2019). Indeed, research from a randomized controlled trial suggests that vaccination acceptability can be improved by including an interactive component in websites, such as an interactive social media component (Daley, Narwaney, Shoup, Wagner, & Glanz, 2018; Glanz et al., 2017). Further research is needed to determine the optimal methods for presenting evidence-based vaccination information on the Internet. Issues concerning vaccination adherence in general are discussed in Chapter 10.

Conclusion

Beliefs, rumors, misinformation, and fear can readily spread through social networks, particularly through social media. The news media can further heighten fears. Researchers and commentators have made various suggestions about how the news media and social media might be reined in, to limit the spread of sensational or inaccurate information. The feasibility and effectiveness of such suggestions remain to be seen. Ultimately, the onus is on the individual to critically examine the sources of information that he or she receives.

CHAPTER 9

IMPROVING RISK COMMUNICATION

Goals of Risk Communication

The purpose of risk communication is to provide the public with the information they need to make well-informed decisions about appropriate actions to take to protect their health and safety. Risk communication should contain more than just tips about good hygiene and the need for vaccination. Ideally, risk communication should contain information about "coping methods, strategies for dealing with stigma, guidance on managing stress when assuming new roles in the family, guidance on building resilience, and psycho-educational materials on grief, anxiety, depression, helplessness, apathy, frustration, anger, and volatility" (Shultz et al., 2008, p. 227).

For risk communication to be effective, the information must be perceived as credible and presented in such a way as to encourage adherence to the recommendations in the message. Research suggests that people are more likely to adhere to health-related recommendations if the following conditions are met: (1) The person believes that the disease is severe and that the recommended behaviors are effective in reducing the risk of infection; (2) the person is worried about contracting the disease and believes that they are susceptible to infection; (3) health authorities are perceived as trustworthy and provide clear, sufficient information; (4) there are few perceived barriers to implementing the recommended health behaviors (Kanadiya & Sallar, 2011).

As we saw earlier, nonadherence to advice from health authorities is a widespread problem. This includes problems with nonadherence to vaccination, hygiene, and social distancing. The topic of risk communication specifically for vaccination is addressed in the following chapter. In the present chapter, we focus on general issues in risk communication, and consider how risk communication might be improved for the next pandemic.

Logical versus Emotional Appeals

Efforts to persuade people to adopt particular behaviors, such as to adopt hygienic practices or to seek vaccination, can involve logical or emotional appeals. Logical appeals refer to facts and statistics, whereas emotional appeals aim to evoke emotion to motivate change (Kim & Choi, 2017). To elicit the desired emotion, emotional appeal messages often include vivid, concrete, image-evoking, and personal elements (Slovic, Finucane, Peters, & MacGregor, 2004). People are more likely to be swayed in their opinions if they are presented with vivid narratives or case examples, as compared to bland statistics about risk (Haase, Betsch, & Renkewitz, 2015). Research indicates that emotional appeals, compared to logical appeals, are more memorable and more likely to stimulate people to seek out health-related information (Betsch, Ulshöfer, Renkewitz, & Betsch, 2011; Janssen, van Osch, de Vries, & Lechner, 2013; Kim & Choi, 2017). Emotional appeals appear to exert their power because induced emotions such as fear are used by people as cues for estimating risk (Slovic, Finucane, Peters, & MacGregor, 2007). Thus, an emotional appeal that elicits fear will tend to increase the person's perceived risk of a particular hazard. But is this the best way to induce adaptive behaviors?

Promoting Adherence by Evoking Fear?

Frightening people into changing their behaviors is a widely used tactic in health promotion campaigns (Muthusamy, Levine, & Weber, 2009). A concern is that such messages might induce widespread anxiety, which can create problems of its own. Some commentators have argued that risk communications should contain a balance of assuring and fear-inducing information (Nerlich & Halliday, 2007). Other commentators have argued that the public should be presented with worst-case scenarios. According to Sandman (2009), a risk-communication consultant, the government must help the public to "visualize what a bad pandemic might be like" (p. 322). Regarding the 2009 Swine flu pandemic, Sandman asserted that "the CDC's biggest failure [was] in not doing enough to help people visualize what a bad pandemic might be like so they can understand and start preparing for the worst" (p. 322).

> [A] reason for the wariness of officials is a fear of being seen to overreact. Critics are already accusing officials of over-warning the

> public, and if the virus recedes and a pandemic never materializes, these critics will consider themselves proved right — as if the fact that your house didn't burn down this year proved the foolishness of last year's decision to buy insurance against fire. (Sandman, 2009, p. 323)

Preparations recommended by Sandman include stocking up on food, water, prescription medicines, and other key supplies. Sandman's (2009) points are that, in terms of preparedness planning: (1) People need to be educated as to how they can protect themselves rather than being treated as passive individuals who have little to do except wash their hands and use facemasks, and (2) people need to err on the side of caution.

> Fundamentally, officials need to ask themselves whether they see the public as potential victims to be protected and reassured, like young children, or as pandemic fighters—grown-ups—who can play an active part in the crisis that might be ahead. ... Having things to do gives people a sense of control. It builds confidence, and it makes them more able to bear their fear. ...... Urging people to prepare can calm those whose concern is excessive and rouse those whose concern is insufficient. (Sandman, 2009, p. 323)

Fear appeals, such as those made in media announcements, and those recommended by Sandman (2009), can be effective in achieving persuasive goals, but their effectiveness depends on a variety of factors, including features of the message and the target audience (Muthusamy et al., 2009; Witte & Allen, 2000). Important factors include the severity of the perceived threat (i.e., perceived severity and personal susceptibility) in relation to what the person believes can be done to cope with the threat (i.e., perceived efficacy) (de Hoog, Stroebe, & de Wit, 2007; Witte, 1992).

Adherence to the guidelines presented in a fear-evoking message is expected to occur if (1) the threat is perceived as severe, (2) an effective coping response is perceived to be available, and (3) the person believes they are capable of executing an effective coping response (Peters, Ruiter, & Kok, 2013). Points (2) and (3) refer to perceived efficacy. When threat is high but perceived efficacy is low, defensive reactions are likely, such as denying the severity of, or susceptibility to, the threat (e.g., disparaging government health warnings) (Goldenberg & Arndt, 2008). The risk needs to be perceived as credible (i.e., not over- or understated) and the preventive or protective measures also need to be perceived as credible. Research suggests that fear appeals are most likely to be effective in promoting health behaviors if (1) the threat is perceived as high *and* (2) efficacy is also perceived as high (Peters et al., 2013).

Fear appeals can sometimes be counterproductive. Telling people that they are at risk of contracting a disease increases their vigilance to disease cues (Duncan & Schaller, 2009; Park et al., 2003, 2007). On the one hand, this can increase the chances of correctly identifying infection and taking appropriate action, such as staying at home so as to prevent spreading disease to others. But on the other hand, it increases the chance that people will misinterpret benign bodily sensations as indications of disease and therefore become unduly anxious and needlessly seeking medical attention and potentially over-taxing the healthcare system. Fear-evoking messages need to be crafted with this issue in mind.

The distinction between monitoring and blunting (Chapter 5) also has implications for the use of fear-evoking messages. People who are monitors, compared to those who are blunters, are more sensitive to fear-evoking messages; that is, their appraisals of risk are more strongly influenced by these messages and they are more likely to remember them (Kim & Choi, 2017). Monitors and blunters do not appear to differ in the impact of logical appeals on risk perception (Kim & Choi, 2017). The research by Kim and Choi suggests that when targeting monitors, fear-evoking messages would be most effective in conveying the seriousness of the risk. In contrast, blunters are likely to distract themselves from such messages. Blunters may benefit from messages that involve logical appeals, which are less likely to trigger avoidance than fear-evoking messages. This suggests that community-wide risk communication programs should consider circulating more than one type of message, with different messages targeting different groups of people such as monitors and blunters.

Psychological Distance Influences Perceived Risk

The concept of psychological distance refers to the perceived distance between the self and an object or experience. For a given health threat (e.g., a particular virus), the shorter the perceived psychological distance, the greater is the perceived threat (and the greater are the odds of triggering the behavioral immune system). Psychological distance varies along four key dimensions (Trope & Liberman, 2010; White et al., 2014):

1. *Spatial distance*. That is, the physical proximity of the disease threat to the person.

2. *Temporal distance*. This refers to two temporal parameters: How soon the threat might arrive, and the temporal origin or newness of the threat. More recently discovered diseases (e.g., the virus causing SARS) tend to be perceived as more dangerous, compared to diseases that have long been present (e.g., viruses causing seasonal influenza), because the former are novel and their pathophysiology may be unknown or unclear (White et al., 2014).

3. *Social distance*. This is defined by the nature of social relationships. People may be more likely to contract pathogens from people who are socially close to them, because they are more frequently in contact (White et al., 2014). A cue to social closeness is the name of the disease. Consistent with this, White et al.'s research indicated that virus names that referenced socially close targets (humans) were perceived as more dangerous by the lay public than diseases that referenced socially distant targets (animals).

4. *Probability distance*: This refers to the chance of encountering an infectious agent, which is determined by factors such as the agent's prevalence in the environment. The perceived probability of an event is influenced by a range of factors, including the cognitive process known as the availability heuristic (Tversky & Kahneman, 1973). That is, the greater the ease of recalling something (e.g., recalling that a given disease has arisen in the community), the greater is its perceived probability of occurring in the future. Consistent with this, research conducted by White et al. (2014) found that the frequency with which a person encounters a virus's name was associated with greater perceived danger.

The concept and findings concerning psychological distance have important implications for risk communication in the media. Health authorities and news agencies must be careful in how—and how often—they publicly discuss disease outbreaks because cues of psychological distance can, on the one hand, lead to undue anxiety or, on the other hand, negatively influence healthcare decisions such as the willingness to seek vaccination (White et al., 2014). Continuous reporting on novel diseases and the repetition of their names may artificially increase perceptions of danger, at least in the short term.

If the goal is to frighten people into adopting health behaviors, then public announcements could emphasize that infection is close at hand, looming in terms of time to impact, and that people have a high probability of infection unless precautionary measures are taken.

Infections that are described as novel (i.e., having newly arisen or newly spread to humans), named after humans (e.g., Asian flu), and continuously reported in the media (i.e., the availability heuristic), will increase the perceived threat of infection. But there are several problems with increasing risk by these means. First, such an approach might undermine the credibility of the risk communication message because some people might think the risks are exaggerated. Second, such messages might truly exaggerate the risk, thereby leading to excessive distress and needless protective behaviors (e.g., needlessly stockpiling food or medication). The naming of outbreaks after humans also runs the risk of leading to discrimination against groups of people, as discussed earlier.

Timing and repetition of risk communication messages are important. People may be initially diligent to adherence to health recommendations but become lax over time. This has been dubbed "flu fatigue" (Levi et al., 2010), which is a form of mass media fatigue described earlier in this volume. Unduly prolonged warning of a future pandemic can lead to flu fatigue in the public (Li et al., 2014; Liao, Cowling, Lam, & Fielding, 2011). Further research is needed to determine the optimal frequency and spacing of messages so as to reduce the chances of flu fatigue.

Managing Rumors

Risk communication is important in the management of rumors. Widespread rumors, including widely disseminated fake news, should not be ignored by health authorities, and if the rumors are true they should be confirmed quickly, along with a factual description of the situation or incident. Rumor surveillance by health authorities is important for the early detection and correction of misinformation and misunderstanding. In such surveillance, healthcare authorities need to actively monitor rumors and misinformation in news media reports and social media. Effective refutation of false rumors reduce uncertainty by offering a clear, point-by-point refutation with solid evidence (DiFonzo & Bordia, 2007). The person or agency doing the refuting should ideally be a trusted party and explain the context in which the refutation is being issued.

Because rumors are sometimes sensational and therefore potentially newsworthy, the news media often contribute to the spreading of rumors (Rosnow & Fine, 1976). And yet, the news media are indispensable for providing the public with information that refutes unfounded rumors (DiFonzo & Bordia, 2007). An unintended and perhaps unavoidable side effect of rumor refutation initiatives is that formal efforts to debunk rumors may, in fact, communicate rumors to people who have not yet heard them.

What can members of the general public do to prevent their perceptions from being biased by rumors circulated by the news media and in the social media? One option is to limit one's exposure to news coverage, to avoid sensational sources, and to give more credence to warnings and advice available from the websites of health authorities such as the WHO and CDC. Warnings and unsubstantiated rumors forwarded from friends or colleagues should be regarded with skepticism.

Conclusion

Several recommendations for effective risk communication were examined in this chapter. Although backed by varying degrees of evidence, even seemingly effective risk communication strategies can backfire under certain conditions. As we saw earlier in this book, the cognitive coping style of monitoring versus blunting can influence a person's receptivity to risk communication. The risk communication recommendations the evoke fear might work for people who have a monitoring cognitive style, but might not be as effective for people who have a blunting cognitive style and therefore are likely to tune out such messages. For people with a blunting cognitive style, other forms of risk communication may be more effective.

Risk communication and programs involving community adherence also need to be conducted with cultural sensitivity in mind. This includes things like training risk communication staff in cultural competency, distributing information in various languages, and involving cultural community leaders in the planning and dissemination of information.

More research is needed to determine the optimal format for pandemic-related risk communication messages. For example, if fear-evoking messages are used, then how can the messages be crafted so as to limit the likelihood of people misinterpreting benign bodily changes or sensations? This is an important issue because misinterpretations can lead to undue anxiety and needless medical consultations, thereby placing undue burden on the healthcare system.

Research is also needed to evaluate the effectiveness of risk communication on people who adhere to conspiracy theories. Do such people tend to reject fear-evoking messages? In the following chapter we will conduct a more detailed examination of the role of attitudinal factors, with a particular emphasis on the important issue of vaccination adherence.

CHAPTER 10

IMPROVING VACCINATION ADHERENCE

Negative Beliefs about Vaccination

Vaccination plays a vital role in managing seasonal influenza and may play an important role in managing the next influenza pandemic. A person's decision to be vaccinated diminishes not only their own risk of infection but also reduces the risk to people with whom they interact. Conversely, anti-vaccination attitudes can contribute to the spread of infection. To illustrate the latter, in December 2014 there was a large outbreak of measles—over 500 cases—centered around Disneyland in Anaheim, California (Zipprich et al., 2015). The outbreak was attributed to parental anti-vaccination beliefs (Haase et al., 2015). Later outbreaks of measles have similarly been attributed to the failure of parents to vaccinate their children (e.g., Lambert, 2019).

The reluctance or frank refusal to have oneself or one's dependents vaccinated—euphemistically known as "vaccine hesitancy"—has been identified by the WHO (2019) as one of the top ten global health threats. People who are vaccination hesitant express concerns about the value or safety of vaccination (Yaqub, Castle-Clarke, Sevdalis, & Chataway, 2014). A review of the literature suggests that hesitant attitudes toward vaccination are widespread and possibly increasing in recent years (Yaqub et al., 2014). Yaqub and colleagues noted that healthcare professionals report increasing challenges in building trustful relationships with patients concerning vaccination, through which they might otherwise allay concerns and assure hesitant patients.

Vaccination hesitancy among HCWs is also growing problem (Maltezou, Theodoridou, Ledda, Rapisarda, & Theodoridou, 2018). Research suggests that fewer than 50% of HCWs, including those involved in direct patient contact, get vaccinated (Antommaria & Prows, 2018; Gruben, Siemieniuk, & McGeer, 2014; Knowler, Barrett, & Watson, 2018). Even during the 2009 Swine flu pandemic, many HCWs were unvaccinated. At a 1,000-bed hospital in Switzerland, for example, only 52% of HCWs were vaccinated (Dorribo, Lazor-Blanchet, Hugli, & Zanetti, 2015).

Conventional programs for improving vaccination rates include public education about the importance of vaccination along with making vaccination easy to obtain and affordable (Levi et al., 2010). Despite these programs, many people fail to seek vaccination. In terms of influenza, people are unlikely to seek vaccination if they (1) believe (accurately or not) that they are unlikely to be exposed to an influenza virus, (2) see themselves as being impervious to infection, (3) do not perceive the infection to be a serious problem, (4) perceive that there are significant inconveniences or barriers to adherence, and (5) have misgivings about the safety and efficacy of vaccination (Ashbaugh et al., 2013; Betsch et al., 2018; Brewer et al., 2007; Holmes, Hughes, & Morrison, 2014; Setbon & Raude, 2010; Yaqub et al., 2014). People with very strong beliefs about negative side effects may refuse to be vaccinated even though they might also acknowledge that the infection is potentially dangerous (Ashbaugh et al., 2013).

Remarkably, many people believe that vaccinations are ineffective or that the risks outweigh the benefits (Betsch et al., 2018; Setbon & Raude, 2010). According to one American survey, a sizable minority (9%) believed that vaccines are more dangerous than the diseases they are supposed to prevent (Newport, 2015). Other surveys have reported even higher figures. In a study conducted in Switzerland during the 2009 Swine flu pandemic, almost half (49%) of the respondents did not think the vaccine would be useful, and most (72%) thought the vaccine could have potentially harmful side effects (Bangerter et al., 2012). In a survey of US college students conducted during the early stage of the same pandemic, only 34% believed that the vaccine was safe (Kanadiya & Sallar, 2011). Research conducted in Canada during the same period found that the decision to not seek vaccination was associated with negative beliefs about the vaccine, such as beliefs about negative side effects (Ashbaugh et al., 2013). Some people refuse vaccination because of beliefs that vaccines are unhealthy because they are "unnatural" (Biss, 2014). According to one poll, more than 20% of US respondents believed that there is a link between childhood vaccination and autism (Public Policy Polling, 2013) even though this claim has been debunked (see Chapter 2). The reasons for HCWs refusing vaccination tend to be similar to those mentioned above (Pless, McLennan, Nicca, Shaw, & Elger, 2017).

Factors Contributing to Vaccination Hesitancy

Aversive past experiences with vaccination may contribute to vaccination hesitancy. Other factors are also important. People with high levels of negative emotionality tend to misinterpret common symptoms or bodily sensations as negative effects of vaccination; that is, the nocebo effect (Data-Franco & Berk, 2013; Petrie et al., 2004). People with high PVD, compared to those with lower levels of PVD, are more likely to engage in hygienic practices such as handwashing (Karademas, Bati, Karkania, Georgiou, & Sofokleous, 2013). Paradoxically, people with high PVD also tend to have negative attitudes towards vaccination (Clay, 2017; Clifford & Wendell, 2016; Hornsey et al., 2018). In other words, heightened aversion to perceived sources of disease predicts more negative attitudes toward vaccines. Clay (2017) offered an evolutionary explanation for the findings: Vaccines have: (1) only recently become a feature of the human environment, (2) are typically administered via common routes of pathogenic transmission (e.g., skin puncture), and (3) intentionally trigger a biological immune response, which is something the BIS aims to minimize.

Belief in conspiracy theories is also associated with vaccination refusal (Cassady et al., 2012; Hornsey et al., 2018). Even exposure to conspiracy theories can cause increase a person's reluctance to seek vaccination (Jolley & Douglas, 2014). Relatedly, mistrust of health authorities is also associated with negative attitudes toward vaccination (Bangerter et al., 2012; Gilles et al., 2011; Yaqub et al., 2014).

Psychological reactance may also play a role in vaccination nonadherence. Psychological reactance is a motivational response to rules, regulations, or attempts at persuasion that are perceived as threatening one's autonomy and freedom of choice (Brehm, 1966; Rosenberg & Siegel, 2017). The perceived threat motivates the person to assert their freedom by rejecting attempts at persuasion, rules, regulation, and other means of control. People vary in the degree to which they are prone to reactance. For a person prone to intense reactance, attempts at persuading them to accept a particular view can paradoxically strengthen their beliefs against the view. A person might endorse anti-science beliefs in an attempt to establish their self-image as a nonconformist; that is, as someone skeptical of consensus views and intolerant of people telling them what to think. Thus, a message that threatens the person's freedom—such as a health warning to get immunized—can induce psychological reactance, which in turn can motivate the person to restore freedom by such means as derogating the source or by adopting a position that is the opposite of that advocated in the message (Brehm & Brehm, 1981; Rains, 2013). Consistent with this, Hornsey et al. (2018) found that people who scored high on a measure of psychological reactance were less likely to seek vaccination.

Changing Vaccination Attitudes

Public education is the typical method used to improve vaccination adherence (CDC, 2018b), and sometimes simple information and assurance about vaccine safety and efficacy suffice to improve adherence. However, this is not always the case. Messages emphasizing the severity of pandemic influenza and the benefits of vaccination sometimes fail to be persuasive (Godinho et al., 2016), for reasons discussed in this and the previous chapter. Myth-busting messages in favor of vaccination can even lead to a paradoxical strengthening of anti-vaccination attitudes in people with high levels of psychological reactance and in people who subscribe to conspiracy theories (Hornsey et al., 2018).

An alternative approach is to target the person's motivations for not seeking vaccination. That is, targeting factors such as psychological reactance, conspiratorial thinking, and PVD. Hornsey and colleagues (Hornsey & Fielding, 2017; Hornsey et al., 2018) offer several practical suggestions for improving vaccination adherence in people who have high levels of psychological reactance and hold anti-vaccination attitudes. These methods are derived from motivational interviewing (Chapter 7) and involve working with people's underlying worldviews; for example, to acknowledge the possibility of conspiracies, but to show how vested interests can conspire to obscure the benefits of vaccination and to exaggerate the dangers. Anti-vaccination movements are high-pressure, highly conformist organizations in which dissenting views are discouraged. To the extent that people reject science because they wish to present a self-image as critical and skeptical, it can be useful to communicate to them the inherently skeptical nature of science and to portray antiscientific thinking as an example of unthinking conformity (Hornsey & Fielding, 2017).

People with high levels of PVD are reluctant to seek vaccination, as discussed earlier, and tend to be conformist in their attitudes (Murray & Schaller, 2012; Murray & Schaller, 2016; Wu & Chang, 2012). Such people may be particularly susceptible to anti-vaccination rhetoric. People with high levels of PVD may also be more likely to pursue quack remedies if such remedies are popular within one's reference group. It is unclear as to how PVD is related to the persuasive effects of pro-vaccination educational campaigns. If PVD plays a causal role in vaccination nonadherence, then the odds of vaccination might also be improved by treating PVD with CBT, as discussed in Chapter 6.

These interventions are best suited on an individual or small group basis. The question arises as to how problems such as psychological reactance could be addressed on a wider, community-based level. Regarding reactance, it may be useful to screen for people prone to psychological reactance and tailor informational messages in a way that makes vaccination seem more appealing. Health messages that are loss focused can be effective. That is, messages that warn recipients of the consequences they will face if they fail to engage in a given protective behavior (e.g., "If you're self-employed and you don't get vaccinated, you could lose income if you get sick") (Gibbons, Gerrard, & Pomery, 2004). Hall and colleagues (2017) developed and validated a brief (3-item) questionnaire of reactance in health settings, which could be adapted to assess a person's psychological reactance to pandemic-related warnings. In this questionnaire, the person is asked to rate their responses to the following items on a 5-point scale (1 = strongly disagree, 5 = strongly agree): "This warning is trying to manipulate me," "The health effect on this warning is overblown," "This warning annoys me." Such a scale could be used as a screening measure. Brief interventions based on motivational interviewing (as discussed earlier) could be used to encourage high-reactance individuals to seek vaccination.

Do it for the Herd

Herd immunity refers to indirect protection from infectious disease that occurs when a large proportion of the population becomes immune to infection, which provides a degree of protection to people who are not immune (Fine et al., 2011). This impedes the spread of infection by disrupting the chain of infection; infection is less likely to spread to non-immune people if they are surrounded by more people who are immune. Herd immunity is important because not all people have access to immunization and some people have medical contraindications to receiving a vaccine. The vaccination rate needed to achieve herd immunity depends on various factors, including population density and the transmissibility of the disease.

Herd immunity can be attained (i.e., the collective population becomes essentially immune) when a sufficient proportion of the population is immune. Estimates vary widely, from 13% to over 90%, depending on the type of influenza virus (Plans-Rubio, 2012). It has been proposed that 80% of healthy persons and 90% of high-risk persons (e.g., HCWs) should be vaccinated (Plans-Rubio, 2012). Although complete herd immunity may be an unattainable goal, methods of boosting the vaccination rate should have a beneficial impact in stemming the spread of infection.

It may be possible to encourage vaccination by appealing to altruistic motives. Many people in the general public are unaware of the importance of herd immunity. For examine, in one survey of 554 American adults, 37% were unfamiliar with the concept of herd immunity, and those unfamiliar with the concept were less likely to seek influenza vaccination (Logan et al., 2018). Public education programs have typically neglected to inform people about herd immunity. Programs are needed to educate people about (1) the concept of herd immunity, (2) the benefits to people who are unable to be vaccinated (i.e., appealing to altruistic motives), and (3) the social undesirability of being a "free rider" (i.e., someone who fails to get vaccinated even though they are medically fit to receive a vaccine). One promotional campaign used the slogan "Do it for the herd" to promote free influenza vaccination (Logan et al., 2018).

A growing body of research suggests that educating people about the collective benefits of vaccination can improve actual herd immunity by increasing the number of people who seek vaccination (Arnesen, Bærøe, Cappelen, & Carlsen, 2018; Böhm, Meier, Groß, Korn, & Betsch, 2018; Hakim et al., 2019; Logan et al., 2018; Vietri et al., 2011). Thus, raising a person's concerns for other people can influence the decision to be vaccinated, providing that people have trust in the health authority's claims about the efficacy and safety of vaccination (Arnesen et al., 2018). There are web-based informational programs about herd immunity, but little is known about their efficacy (Hakim et al., 2019). These web-based representations show people what herd immunity is, and how it is achieved.

Targeting Superspreaders

Recall from Chapter 1 that superspreaders are people who disproportionately contribute to the spreading of infection. Obvious ways of reducing superspreading are to encourage people to seek vaccination and perform basic hygiene, and to encourage infected people to stay at home and away from public places (including hospitals) if they are contagious. To this end, hospitals often have signs posted advising people to not visit hospitals if they are suffering from flu-like symptoms.

It has been argued that vaccination programs that specifically target superspreaders are likely to be more effective than indiscriminate mass vaccination programs (Lloyd-Smith, Schreiber, Kopp, & Getz, 2005; Skene, Paltiel, Shim, & Galvani, 2014). This is because, by definition, superspreaders, compared to the general population, have a greater impact on the spread of infection. The concept of targeted vaccination raises questions about how such people could be identified and how they might be specifically encouraged to seek vaccination. Proxy measures could be used to identify people who have a strong potential for superspreading, such as persons who have high levels of contact with other people. In terms of pandemic management, if an effective vaccine is available, it may prove useful to strongly encourage vaccination for people who work at jobs in which they have high levels of contact with the general public (e.g., hospitality industry workers), or frequent contact with the medically frail (e.g., HCWs). Administration of vaccines to high-contact people might involve vaccination at schools, workplaces, and at public venues (Skene et al., 2014).

Little is known about the possible benefits of public education campaigns that specifically discuss the topic of superspreading. Such campaigns could educate the public about the concept of superspreading and provide advice about how to avoid superspreading. Such a campaign could include simple statements such as "Don't be a superspreader: Prevent the spread of infection by getting vaccinated, being hygienic, and staying away from public places if you have flu-like symptoms." The potential benefits of such a campaign remain to be investigated.

Treating Injection Phobia

Although people may avoid vaccinations for various attitudinal reasons, as discussed earlier (e.g., safety concerns, distrust of health authorities), some people avoid vaccinations primarily because of fear of injections (Yaqub et al., 2014). Indeed, people with injection phobia tend to avoid vaccinations (Ritz et al., 2014). According to one survey of 883 adults and 1,024 children, sampled from the general population, fear of injections was the primary reason for immunization refusal in 7% of adults and 8% of children (Taddio et al., 2012). Even 10% of HCWs in roles involving direct patient contact avoided vaccination because of an aversion to injections (Knowler et al., 2018). Accordingly, vaccination adherence during times of pandemic may be improved by treating injection phobia.

Injection phobia—also known by the more cumbersome diagnostic label, blood-injury-injection phobia—refers to a severe (i.e., impairing) fear and avoidance of injections (American Psychiatric Association, 2013). People who have injection phobia typically fear and avoid stimuli associated with blood or injury. In many cases of injection phobia, the person may become lightheaded and faint when exposed to injections or to stimuli associated with blood or injury. The person may feel faint, turn pale, and start to sweat and tremble, and in some cases may lose consciousness. These episodes usually resolve within minutes although there is a risk of embarrassment and injuries from falls. People with injection phobia may fear and avoid the fainting reaction, or they may have a strong fear and avoidance of the pain associated with injections (American Psychiatric Association, 2013; Ritz, Meuret, & Alvord, 2014). Anticipatory anxiety is a feature of injection phobia and phobias in general (Barlow, 2004). Indeed, sometimes the most distressing aspect of injection phobia is the worry or anxiety that occurs before a person is scheduled to receive an injection, which can motivate the person to avoid or flee.

Various methods can be used to treat injection phobia. Distraction at the time of injection is commonly implemented by people who administer injections, with some evidence of efficacy (Birnie, Noel, Chambers, Uman, & Parker, 2018; Riddell, Taddio, McMurtry, Chambers et al., 2015). For example, asking patients to imagine some pleasant event (e.g., asking them to describe their last vacation), video or music distraction, deep breathing exercises, or asking patients (e.g., children) to focus on some distracting stimuli during the injection (e.g., using props blowing on a pinwheel as they are being injected (e.g., Andrews & Shaw, 2010). One group of HCWs developed a "Vaccination Comfort Menu" (Kuntz et al., 2019), consisting of a poster offering various options for alleviating the distress associated with injections (e.g., offering distractions such as a squeeze ball, pinwheel or headphones).

Although useful, these methods are of limited value for people with severe injection phobia, because such people, due to their strong anticipatory anxiety, avoid attending clinics for injections. In such cases, more intensive interventions may be needed. CBT protocols, such as those employing a method known as applied tension (Öst & Sterner, 1987) can be useful in as few as 1-5 sessions and has demonstrated efficacy in treatment outcome studies (McMurtry et al., 2016; Meuret, Simon, Bhaskara, & Ritz, 2017). Applied tension involves tensing the torso, legs, or non-injected arm during exposure to blood, injury, or injection stimuli, as a means of offsetting the decline in blood pressure (i.e., the fainting or vasovagal reaction) that can occur in injection phobia.

During times of pandemic in which effective vaccinations are available, it is important that people with injection phobia are informed that there are quick, effective ways of treating their phobia and thereby making it easier for them to be vaccinated. Public awareness announcements could provide people with information and resources for coping with injection-related distress. These could include handouts, websites with instructional videos about how to use distracting imagery, and instructional videos devoted to illustrating ways of self-implementing CBT for injection phobia, such as applied tension (Meuret et al., 2017; Riddell, Taddio, McMurtry, Shah et al., 2015).

Is Mandatory Vaccination a Viable Option?

Even if an effective vaccine is available for the next pandemic, it would likely be necessary to provide some sort of incentives for people to seek vaccination. This is because, as we saw earlier in this volume, many people do not seek vaccination during seasonal influenza and even during pandemic influenza. Incentives may come in the form of "nudges"; for example, public service announcements about the importance of "doing it for the herd" by getting vaccinated. Vaccination may also be mandated, although this raises a host of ethical and other issues.

Many clinics or hospitals require HCWs to receive influenza vaccination as a condition of employment (Antommaria & Prows, 2018; Born, Ikura, & Laupacis, 2015). This is important because, as noted earlier, a remarkably high percentage of HCWs fail to seek vaccination, even though they come into contact with medically frail patients, for whom even seasonal influenza could prove lethal. Mandatory vaccination programs have also been implemented in schools and preschools as a condition of enrollment because these settings tend to be hot spots for the spreading of infection (see Chapter 2). Computer simulations suggest that a policy of sending home unvaccinated students can significantly stem the spread of infection (Getz et al., 2016).

The pros and cons of mandatory vaccination programs have been debated extensively in the healthcare literature (e.g., Behrman & Offley, 2013; Born et al., 2015; Lukich, Kekewich, & Roth, 2018). One argument is that mandatory programs unduly infringe on their liberties and right to autonomy. In response, it has been shown that mandatory vaccination programs can be useful in stemming the spread of infection and its effects (Antommaria & Prows, 2018; Born et al., 2015; Frederick et al., 2018; Wang, Jing, & Bocchini, 2017). Accordingly, influenza vaccination should be mandatory for front-line HCWs because these individuals have a duty of care to patients (Cortes-Penfield, 2014; Jones-Berry, 2018). When individuals make the decision to work in the medical field, they are expected to put the safety of their patients ahead of their own interests, and the minimal discomfort that may result from a vaccine is not enough to negate the responsibilities that HCWs have toward their patients (Lukich et al., 2018).

If mandatory vaccination is useful for HCWs and school children, then what about other segments of the population? Should mandatory vaccination be implemented, for example, for people who come into frequent contact with other people, such as workers in the hospitality industry? Some restaurants and food services have required their workers to be vaccinated for Hepatitis A (e.g., EHS Today, 2000). The same could be done for influenza.

For mandatory vaccination programs, people can apply for exemptions under special circumstances, such as on medical grounds. For example, vaccination may be contraindicated in people who have severe allergies to egg proteins, which are contained in some vaccines (Gruenberg & Shaker, 2011). Vaccination may also be refused on religious grounds. In Western countries, the rates of refusal for religious reasons seems unlikely to be high. In a study of over 15,000 Cincinnati hospital employees, for example, found that only 0.08% (n = 12) refused vaccination on religious grounds (Antommaria & Prows, 2018). Most of these refusers identified themselves as Christian and most expressed purity concerns; that is, concerns that the vaccine or its mode of administration was impure, or receiving the vaccine would make the person impure. Two individuals, for example, believed (erroneously) that the influenza vaccine contained cells derived from aborted human fetuses. Although all the exceptions were approved by the hospital, the study pointed to an opportunity to improve vaccination uptake in these refusers. This could be done by correcting misconceptions, and by consulting with religious leaders on issues of whether vaccination is a source of impurity (Antommaria & Prows, 2018).

What proportion of the general population would adhere to mandated but unenforced (and unenforceable?) vaccination? As we saw earlier in this volume, some people react to threats against their autonomy with intense psychological reactance, and as noted earlier in this chapter, some people have strongly held anti-vaccination beliefs. Such individuals are likely to resist any efforts at forcing them to be vaccinated. In comparison, other people are conformists in regard to healthcare in that they are obedient to authority and/or seek approval by adhering to the norms of their peer groups. Multiple factors are at play in shaping conformity versus reactance, and little is known about the prevalence of conformity versus reactance to the guidelines presented by healthcare authorities. However, research shows that the introduction of mandatory vaccination for HCWs leads to an increase in vaccination rate (Antommaria & Prows, 2018; Frederick et al., 2018; Leibu & Maslow, 2015). Barriers to getting vaccinated, such as injection phobia, can be overcome by the methods described earlier.

Attitudes toward mandatory vaccination are not static, they may change over time. Although some people may be initially resistant to the idea of mandatory vaccination, they may come to gradually accept the idea. In North America, most HCWs appear to be in favor of condition-of-service influenza vaccination policies (Gruben et al., 2014), although a small study suggested that mandatory vaccination would not be strongly supported in the UK (Stead et al., 2019). Ultimately, “nudges” or incentives (e.g., in the form of public education programs) may be the optimal way of increasing vaccination adherence in the general population, whereas mandated vaccination—assuming there is an effective vaccine—may be important and even necessary for people such as HCWs and perhaps workers in other sectors.

Conclusion

Vaccination hesitancy is a widespread, important problem, even among HCWs and even during times of pandemic. Various types of negative attitudes and other psychological factors appear to play a role, such as psychological reactance, PVD, and injection phobia. Treating the attitudinal and motivational roots of the problem may be vital during the next pandemic. Public education campaigns show promise as do interventions targeting particular problems such as injection phobia. Mandatory vaccination as a requirement for employment may be viable for HCWs and workers in other sectors. It is unclear whether mandatory vaccination would be viable on a community-wide level.

CHAPTER 11

TREATING PANDEMIC-RELATED EMOTIONAL DISTRESS

A Screen-and-Treat Approach

In the event of disaster such as a pandemic, a lack of mental health and social support systems and a lack of well-trained mental health professionals can increase the risk that people will develop emotional and other forms of psychological disorders (Shultz et al., 2015). A proactive response is required, involving a rapid assessment of outbreak-associated psychological stressors, for both civilians and HCWs. But even at the best of times, busy medical practitioners, such as primary care physicians, often fail to detect psychological disorders (Cano-Vindel et al., 2018; Rubin & Wessely, 2013). The situation is even more challenging during a pandemic, where there is an increase in the number of sick people and likely staff shortages due to illness. Accordingly, there need to be efficient procedures for identifying people who are at risk for, or actually suffering from, clinically significant distress. Procedures are also needed for selecting optimal interventions. The screen-and-treat method is one such approach.

One of the best recent examples of the screen-and-treat approach was one implemented by Brewin and colleagues in the aftermath of the 2005 London terrorist bombings (Brewin et al., 2008). The program, which was designed primarily to treat PTSD, was widely advertised to health professionals and the general public, and treatment was offered free of charge. A dedicated 24-hour helpline was established that provided general advice and to refer callers to a screening team. People contacting the program were screened using validated measures. Those people screening positive were invited to complete a more detailed assessment with a clinician. People with preexisting mental health problems were either referred back to their treatment provider or referred for appropriate treatment. Those people with mental health problems arising since the bombings were assessed for suitability for trauma-focused treatment. The goal was to target cases in which symptoms were likely to be persistent. Based on the self-reported trajectory of symptoms, a clinical decision was made to either refer the patient for immediate treatment or to continue monitoring, with the expectation that the symptoms would resolve with time. For those patients referred for treatment, the intervention consisted primarily of CBT, which led to significant reductions in symptom severity.

This program serves as a model that could be adapted to treat mental health problems arising in the event of a pandemic. Important considerations in adapting such a program are: (1) Limiting the burden on healthcare providers to assess for mental health problems, (2) implementing triaged or stepped-care interventions that are efficient, economically viable to the healthcare system (given other, competing priorities for pandemic control) and readily accessible by large numbers of people, and (3) limiting the risk of infection being spread to the front-line clinicians who would be responsible for assessing and treating mental health problems arising from a pandemic. A flowchart outlining such a program appears in Figure 11-1.

One of the lessons learned from previous outbreaks, such as the Spanish flu and the SARS outbreak, is that patient care can be compromised, sometimes severely so, if healthcare providers become infected. The odds of infection are high if healthcare providers are in continuous face-to-face contact with many potentially sick people. In the next pandemic, much of the assessment and treatment of mental health problems could be conducted by video conferencing, such as through one of the many video conferencing software programs available on the Internet (e.g., Skype™). This is a viable option because most (>56%) of the world's population and most (89%) of the developed world has Internet access (https://www.internetworldstats.com/stats.htm, accessed May 16, 2019).

Figure 11-1. Screen-and-treat flowchart for targeting emotional distress.

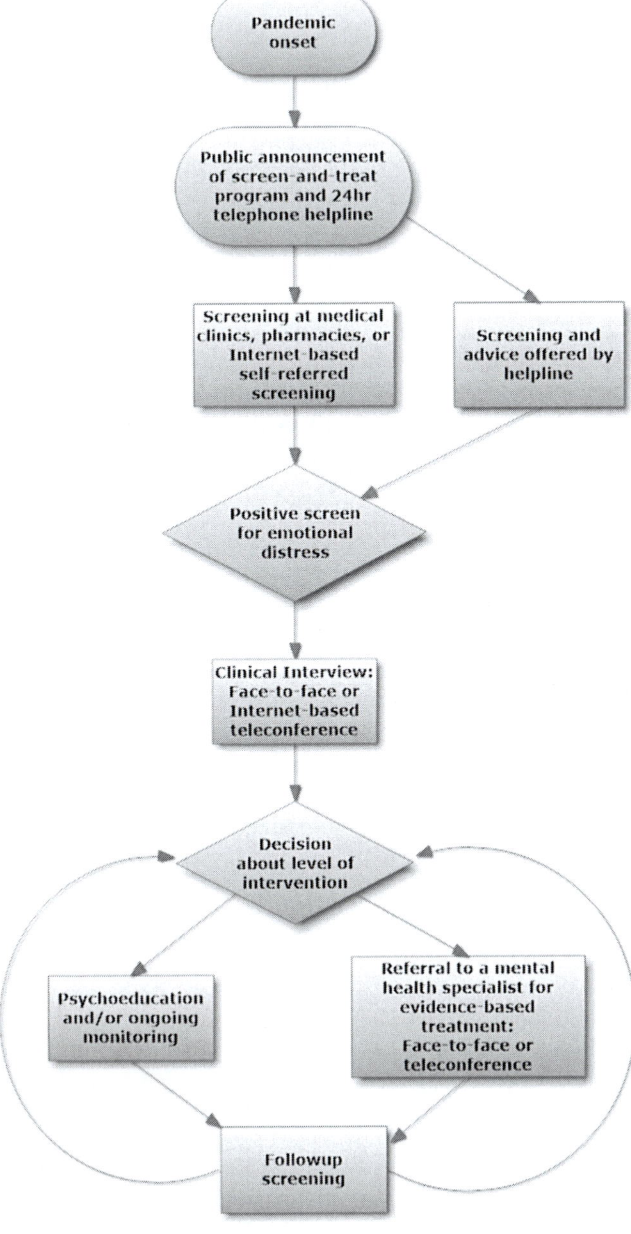

Screening Methods

Brief screening tools for mood and anxiety disorders are important for improving mental healthcare in medical settings, such as in primary care, because HCWs typically do not have the time or training to administer diagnostic interviews. Thus, the use of validated screening instruments is an important first step in integrating care for mood and anxiety disorders into existing primary healthcare services (Ali, Ryan, & De Silva, 2016). Efficient screening is the cornerstone for treating pandemic-related emotional problems. Brief screening instruments have been developed for use in primary health clinics. For example, the 4-item, computer-administered Patient Health Questionnaire-4 has good levels of reliability and validity for assessing depression and general anxiety, and has established cut-off scores for identifying patients in need of a more detailed evaluation (Cano-Vindel et al., 2018). A brief, psychometrically sound screen for PTSD is the 4-item Primary Care PTSD screener (Breslau, Peterson, & Schultz, 2008; Spoont et al., 2015).

An issue for further investigation is whether it is clinically useful to assess maladaptive avoidance. This refers to the avoidance of places, people, or activities that is excessive, given the objective danger, and leads to impairments in functioning. An example is avoiding the workplace even though it is not currently a place of infection and is not considered hazardous by health authorities.

Another question for further investigation concerns the value of screening for vulnerability factors that may lead to pandemic-related distress. People with high levels of PVD, for example, are at heightened risk of becoming distressed during a pandemic. This vulnerability can be measured by the 15-item PVDS. The merits of including this scale in a screening battery remain to be examined.

Interventions for Treating Pandemic-Related Distress

Pandemic-related distress may fade without intervention, just like the emotional effects of other stressors can fade over time (Rubin & Wessely, 2013). Accordingly, people who are merely worried or mildly distressed about a pandemic, without any sign of impaired functioning because of their worry, might be provided with education about how to deal with stress, as described in the following section. For people who experience severe levels of pandemic-related distress, more intensive interventions would be required. Examples of disorders meriting clinical attention include major depressive disorder and PTSD triggered by the loss of loved ones or other traumatic events, and generalized anxiety disorder that may be triggered (or exacerbated) by the uncertainty associated with a pandemic. Such people could be referred for CBT or treatment with particular medications (e.g., selective serotonin reuptake inhibitors). There are various empirically-supported CBT protocols and forms of pharmacotherapy for treating emotional distress (Nathan & Gorman, 2015).

Psychological interventions can be useful in the early stages of a pandemic, when anticipatory anxiety and worry are likely to be high, and in later stages, especially where people are exposed to traumatic events such as witnessing the death of friends and loved ones. Psychological interventions can be useful even after the pandemic has passed. Some people, for example, experience protracted, clinically severe, protracted grief reactions when loved ones die (Mauro et al., 2018). CBT or other empirically supported interventions can help these individuals (Doering & Eisma, 2016; Shear & Gribbin Bloom, 2017). Community memorial services and other symbols of remembrance can also be beneficial in improving social support for people who have lost loved ones.

As we saw in the case of SARS, PTSD can persist well after the infectious epidemic has passed. People with persistent pandemic-related PTSD would likely benefit from empirically supported treatments such as trauma-focused CBT (Taylor, 2017). Therapy could be delivered over the Internet (e.g., via Skype) if severe social distancing restrictions are in place. If quarantine is implemented, people can be prepared to cope with the experience in various ways; for example, by being provided with means of remaining in contact with loved ones (e.g., computer or cellphone access) and being provided with information about the nature and likely duration of quarantine.

Stress Management Advice for the General Public

Several organizations have developed factsheets offering advice about how people can cope with stress during a pandemic (e.g., American Psychological Association, 2004, 2011; American Red Cross, 2009; Canadian Psychological Association, 2009). They include the following recommendations about emotional and physical self-care:

- *Stay informed about how to keep safe.* Seek out information from a credible source such as the WHO or CDC, or a local health agency. Follow the guidelines of public health agencies. This might involve staying at home or avoiding public gatherings. Be wary of unsubstantiated rumors. Remember that the media tend to sensationalize things, such as by focusing on the bad news (e.g., people who become sick) and neglecting the more mundane good news (e.g., the many people who didn't get sick). Limit your exposure to websites or TV programs that fuel your fears.
- *Keep things in perspective.* For centuries people have survived hardships. Most people are resilient; most people bounce back and adapt to changes. Do not dwell on worst-case scenarios. Remember, things will get better.
- *Stay healthy.* A healthy lifestyle, including proper diet, exercise, sleep, and rest, is a good defense against illness. Avoid alcohol and other intoxicating substances. Practicing good hygiene, such as handwashing and covering coughs, will minimize the spread of infection to you and others. Get vaccinated. A healthy body can have a positive impact on your thoughts and emotions, enabling you to make better decisions and help you deal with the flu's uncertainties. Take time to relax. Maintain your normal routine as far as you can.
- *Build resilience.* Resilience is the process of adapting and coping in the face of adversity. Draw on skills that you have successfully used in the past to cope with life's challenges. Use those skills to help manage your concerns about the flu's uncertainties.
- *Have a plan.* Having a plan to cope with hardships can lessen your anxiety. In case health officials recommend that you stay at home, keep at least a two-week supply of non-perishable, easy to prepare food, water, and other important household and other supplies, including medical supplies. Consider options for working from home. Plan for how you might care for sick family members. Establish an emergency family communication plan. Plan on how you might spend your time if schools or businesses are closed. Plan to stay at home if you are ill.
- *Communicate with your children.* Discuss the flu in an open, age-appropriate manner with your children. Address your children's concerns. Remember that children take their cues from adults; if they see that you're upset then they will become upset. As far as

possible, try to maintain your children's routines and schedules. If you do notice that your child's behavior has changed significantly at home or at school, discuss the situation with them.

- *Keep connected.* Maintaining social networks can be a valuable way of sharing feelings and relieving stress. You can stay connected via social media if health authorities recommend that you limit face-to-face social contacts. But remember to take breaks from thinking and talking about stressful things in your life.
- *When to seek help.* Some degree of fear or anxiety about the flu is normal, but sometimes people need help to cope with stress. Look for warning signs such as the following: (1) Persistent anxiety, worry, insomnia, irritability, or depression, (2) avoiding social contacts to the point that you have become isolated, (3) persistently checking one's body (e.g., taking your temperature) or persistently seeking reassurance about your health from doctors, friends, family, or the Internet, (4) engaging in excessive or unnecessary hygiene precautions, such as wearing a facemask at home or repeatedly washing your hands when there is no need to do so, or (5) abusing alcohol or drugs, or overeating, as a way of coping with stress.
- *Where to seek help.* If any of the warning signs apply to you, then you may benefit from seeing a licensed mental health professional such as a psychologist, family physician, or counselor. Sometimes a consultation can be conducted via the Internet. Consulting with a healthcare professional can help you devise a plan for coping with stress.

Helping the Helpers

During the next pandemic, HCWs are likely to experience various kinds of job-related stressors, including (1) a heightened risk of personal infection, sickness, and death, due to their frequent contact with pandemic patients, (2) overwork and fatigue, (3) exposure to the death of others, including exposure to deaths on a mass scale, including the death of children, (4) the inability to save others despite great efforts, (5) threats of violence from people seeking scare or limited medical resources, (6) separation from family, loved ones, and social supports during the pandemic response, and (7) the stress of inadvertently spreading infection to others, including friends, family and loved ones (Gardner & Moallef, 2015; Shultz et al., 2008). Thus, in addition to the interventions discussed earlier in this chapter, it would be useful to provide training to HCWs, such as hospital nursing and medical staff, in the psychological aspects and management of pandemic-related distress. Treatment resources particularly for front-line HCWs would also be useful, such as collaborative pandemic planning and organizational preparedness training, increasing emotional resilience by promoting adaptive coping (training in stress management, encouraging self-care such as taking regular breaks), provision of peer support, identifying those at high risk and providing intervention, and offering long-term support after the event to assist with residual effects (Gardner & Moallef, 2015). For front-line healthcare teams, it would be important to build team cohesion and morale so as to combat fear, helplessness, and burnout (Shultz et al., 2008). HCWs also would likely need support if they or their families being threatened or ostracized because people fear exposure to disease.

Conclusion

A screen-and-treat approach is a promising method for identifying and treating people who suffer from significant pandemic-related distress. This approach has proved successful for treating other forms of community-wide distress although its efficacy for pandemic-related distress remains to be evaluated. Patients with severe psychiatric disorders that are induced or exacerbated by a pandemic might benefit from a combination of CBT and particular medications.

An issue for further research is whether pandemic-related distress should be managed with a symptom-focused approach (i.e., treating cases as they arise) or whether vulnerability factors should be targeted, such as high levels of PVD. The assessment of vulnerability factors might be particularly useful in the early stages of a pandemic, to identify people who are especially likely to experience pandemic-related emotional problems. If high levels of PVD lead to socially disruptive behaviors such as out-group discrimination, as discussed earlier, then reductions in PVD, via CBT, could have beneficial effects at a societal level. These possibilities await further investigation.

CHAPTER 12

GENERAL CONCLUSIONS AND FUTURE DIRECTIONS

A Portrait of the Next Pandemic

Theory, research, and case descriptions described in this book make it possible to sketch a portrait of what things will probably be like during the next pandemic. Dealing with the psychological fallout of a severe pandemic will not be a simple task. Things are likely to be complicated, unpredictable, and turbulent. There will be widespread prosocial behavior but also incidents of civil unrest and even rioting. Other fallouts will include a rise of xenophobia and discrimination. Ethnic minority groups and HCWs will likely be targets of discrimination. We will see a proliferation of conspiracy theories. Someone or some organization or agency will be blamed, rightly or wrongly. The news media will sensationalize the pandemic, despite admonishments to engage in more balanced reporting. Unfounded rumors and fake news will spread rapidly throughout the Internet. Heath authorities will struggle to contain rumors and to debunk conspiracy theories.

Many people will dutifully conform to the advice of health authorities. Such people will get vaccinated, cover their coughs, and comply with social distancing mandates. But many other people will fail to adhere to the recommendations of health authorities. These people will engage in seeming self-defeating behaviors such as refusing to get vaccinated, if a vaccine is available. These people will refuse to stay home when they are sick. They will spread infection to other people.

There will be a rise of quack cures and folk remedies. Charlatans will seize the opportunity to capitalize on mass fears. During the Spanish flu, bicycle vendors sought to promote their wares by claiming that bicycles were good for you, because cycling kept you out in the fresh air, away from the stuffy, contaminated confines of public transportation. Similar claims will likely to be made by unscrupulous entrepreneurs during the next pandemic. There will also be price gouging. As people rush to buy things to protect themselves, such as N95 respirator masks, unscrupulous vendors will raise the prices astronomically.

Schools, places of worship, and other places of congregation will be closed. Portions of the infrastructure such as sanitation services may collapse due to worker absenteeism. People will be advised to remain at home, where their primary source of social connection and social support will be through electronic means, such as the Internet and cellular phones. Many people will cope well with the imposed isolation, especially those with an active presence on social media platforms such as Facebook or Twitter. Other people will experience intense loneliness and boredom as a result of social distancing restrictions.

Hospital emergency departments and other clinics will see a surge of patients, including a multitude of the "worried well." The hospital surge will even occur in places that the pandemic has not yet reached because people will misinterpret minor ills such as coughs or bodily aches as signs of pandemic infection. In places where the pandemic is widespread, hospitals will be unable to accommodate the influx of patients. The sick will be sent home either to fend for themselves or to be cared for by their significant others.

Many people will be resilient to the stressors associated with the pandemic. Many people will stoically accept the risks posed by the pandemic and do their best to protect themselves and their loved ones. But many other people will become highly anxious and frightened. Some people may experience debilitating anxiety that is so severe that it impairs their daily functioning. Such people will try to protect themselves, but in extreme ways such as wearing masks and protective gloves in their homes or apartments, even when they are alone.

Depression and grief will be widespread if there is a significant death toll. If the next pandemic is like some past pandemics in which children and young adults were most susceptible, then there will be many parents grieving for their lost children. If this happens, then the adverse mental health effects of the pandemic could be severe and long-lasting. Mental health consequences of the pandemic, such as PTSD and depression, may persist long after the infection has passed.

People who score high on vulnerability traits, such as negative emotionality, intolerance of uncertainty, and PVD, are likely to become particularly distressed during the pandemic. Ideally, screening programs would be available, such as screening with the PVDS or short measures of anxiety or depression, to identify people in need of mental health services. Such services could be delivered over the Internet so as to reduce unnecessary face-to-face contacts.

There will be widespread uncertainty after the pandemic has passed. For some time after, people will wonder whether the pandemic has truly passed or whether the next wave is about to arrive. People with particular vulnerability factors, such as high level of intolerance of uncertainty or overestimation of threat, will continue to worry long after the threat has passed. Such people would benefit from psychological interventions such as CBT.

Managing Future Pandemics

For the next pandemic, the current recommendations of organizations like the WHO and CDC, as discussed throughout this volume, will be insufficient. There are three interrelated sets of important needs that are not adequately addressed in current, conventional methods for managing pandemics: (1) The need for improving risk communication, (2) the need for improving adherence regarding health-promoting behaviors (e.g., vaccination), and (3) the need for addressing mental health issues such as the emergence or worsening of emotional problems. Throughout this volume, we have considered various ways of addressing these issues.

Two main types of psychosocial interventions were discussed in this book: (1) Health promotion strategies to facilitate adherence to vaccination, hygiene, and social distancing programs; and (2) interventions that are part of a screen-and-treat approach for treating mental health problems. Both types of interventions should be implemented within the context of a broader management strategy that targets the global health and well-being of people and their communities. The interventions discussed in this volume have their place within the broader guidelines for helping people deal with large-scale emergencies, such as the guidelines provided by the Inter-Agency Standing Committee (2007) for offering mental health and social support in emergency settings. This committee provides a means of coordinating humanitarian assistance among key United Nations programs and other assistance programs. Four levels of intervention have been proposed by the committee for dealing with mental health and social support in emergency settings: (1) Restoring basic services and security for the affected population, (2) strengthening family and community networks, (3) providing distressed individuals with social support, and (4) providing specialized mental health intervention for severely affected survivors. The present volume has focused largely on the latter two levels of intervention.

A Roadmap for Future Research

There are several important directions for future research to better understand the psychology of pandemics. A better understanding of why people do or do not adhere to health recommendations has important implications for how health authorities educate the public and implement interventions for curbing the spread of infection. Research is needed to refine and evaluate methods for improving adherence to hygiene, vaccination, and social distancing programs. Relatedly, negative attitudes toward vaccination is an important issue in managing pandemics. A deeper understanding of the motivational roots of these negative attitudes is important. As we saw in this volume, several factors are associated with such attitudes, including PVD, the tendency to believe in conspiracy theories, and psychological reactance.

A new generation of studies is required to find ways of improving adherence to vaccination and hygiene. Recent novel research suggests some ways in which hygiene adherence might be improved. For example, visual cues can be useful, such as automated towel dispensers in public washrooms set to present a towel either with or without activation by users (Ford, Boyer, Menachemi, & Huerta, 2014). Building on the assumption that hand hygiene behavior is socially desirable, Pfattheicher and colleagues (2018) found that handwashing in public toilets was improved when stylized eyes were added to health signs advising that handwashing protects against the spread of pathogens. The replicability of such novel findings needs to be established. Nevertheless, the studies illustrate how psychological research is relevant to improving adherence to hygiene behaviors.

Research on optimal methods of screening for, and treating pandemic-related distress is also warranted, including the development and testing of reliable, efficient methods for identifying people at greatest risk of developing pandemic-related psychopathology. Another issue is whether it is feasible to develop community-wide methods for reducing xenophobia and other forms of discrimination that occur when people are threatened with infection. Most of the findings and health promotion programs discussed in this volume come from the Western world and, to some extent, from Asia and Africa. Further research is needed to determine whether the findings can be generalized to other regions, including places in the developing world that have not been investigated.

REFERENCES

Aarøe, L., Petersen, M. B., & Arceneaux, K. (2017). The behavioral immune system shapes political intuitions: Why and how individual differences in disgust sensitivity underlie opposition to immigration. *American Political Science Review, 111*, 277-294. doi:10.1017/S0003055416000770

Abeysinghe, S., & White, K. (2010). Framing disease: The avian influenza pandemic in Australia. *Health Sociology Review, 19*, 369-381. doi:10.5172/hesr.2010.19.3.369

Abramowitz, J. S., & Braddock, A. E. (2011). *Hypchondriasis and health anxiety*. Cambridge, MA: Hogrefe & Huber.

Ackerman, J. M., Hill, S. E., & Murray, D. R. (2018). The behavioral immune system: Current concerns and future directions. *Social and Personality Psychology Compass, 12*, 57-70. doi:10.1111/spc3.12371

Adebayo, G., Neumark, Y., Gesser-Edelsburg, A., Abu Ahmad, W., & Levine, H. (2017). Zika pandemic online trends, incidence and health risk communication: A time trend study. *BMJ Global Health, 2*, e000296. doi:10.1136/bmjgh-2017-000296

Aiello, A. E., Coulborn, R. M., Aragon, T. J., Baker, M. G., Burrus, B. B., Cowling, B. J., . . . Vukotich, C. J. (2010). Research findings from nonpharmaceutical intervention studies for pandemic influenza and current gaps in the research. *American Journal of Infection Control, 38*, 251-258.

Al-Tawfiq, J. A., & Memish, Z. A. (2016). Drivers of MERS-CoV transmission: What do we know? *Expert Review of Respiratory Medicine, 10*, 331-338. doi:10.1586/17476348.2016.1150784

Alcalde-Cabero, E., Almazán-Isla, J., López, F. J. G., Ara-Callizo, J. R., Avellanal, F., Casasnovas, C., . . . de Pedro-Cuesta, J. (2016). Guillain-Barré syndrome following the 2009 pandemic monovalent and seasonal trivalent influenza vaccination campaigns in Spain from 2009 to 2011: Outcomes from active surveillance by a neurologist network, and records from a country-wide hospital discharge database. *BMC Neurology, 16*, article 75. doi:10.1186/s12883-016-0598-z

Ali, G.-C., Ryan, G., & De Silva, M. J. (2016). Validated screening tools for common mental disorders in low and middle income countries: A systematic review. *PLoS ONE, 11,* article e0156939. doi:10.1371/journal.pone.0156939

Allport, G., & Postman, L. (1947). *The psychology of rumor.* New York: Holt.

American Psychiatric Association. (2000). *Diagnostic and statistical manual of mental disorders (4th ed., text rev.).* Washington, DC: Author.

American Psychiatric Association. (2013). *Diagnostic and statistical manual of mental disorders (5th ed.).* Arlington, VA: Author.

American Psychological Association. (2004). The road to resilience, http://www. apahelpcenter.org/featuredtopics/feature. php?id=6, accessed April 26, 2019.

American Psychological Association. (2011). Managing your anxiety about H1N1 flu (swine flu), https://www.apa.org/helpcenter/h1n1-flu, accessed April 5, 2019.

American Red Cross. (2009). Preparing for a swine flu (H1N1) pandemic, http://georgiadisaster.info/flu/Red%20Cross%20Fllu%20Preparedness.pdf, accessed April 5, 2019.

Andrews, G. J., & Shaw, D. (2010). "So we started talking about a beach in Barbados": Visualization practices and needle phobia. *Social Science & Medicine, 71,* 1804-1810. doi:10.1016/j.socscimed.2010.08.010

Antommaria, A. H., & Prows, C. A. (2018). Content analysis of requests for religious exemptions from a mandatory influenza vaccination program for healthcare personnel. *Journal of Medical Ethics, 44,* 389-391. doi:10.1136/medethics-2017-104271

Antonelli, M., & Donelli, D. (2018). Reinterpreting homoeopathy in the light of placebo effects to manage patients who seek homoeopathic care: A systematic review. *Health & Social Care in the Community.* doi:10.1111/hsc.12681

Ariely, D. (2014). *Predictably irrational: The hidden forces that shape our decisions.* New York: HarperCollins.

Arnesen, S., Bærøe, K., Cappelen, C., & Carlsen, B. (2018). Could information about herd immunity help us achieve herd immunity? Evidence from a population representative survey experiment. *Scandinavian Journal of Public Health, 46,* 854-858. doi:10.1177/1403494818770298

Arnold, C. (2018a). "Eat more onions!": Desperate and massively debatable medical advice from 1918. *Lapham's Quarterly, https://www.laphamsquarterly.org/roundtable/eat-more-onions,* accessed January 25, 2019.

Arnold, C. (2018b). *Pandemic 1918: Eyewitness accounts from the greatest medical holocaust in modern history*. New York: St. Martin's Press.

Ashbaugh, A. R., Herbert, C. F., Saimon, E., Azoulay, N., Olivera- Figueroa, L., & Brunet, A. (2013). The decision to vaccinate or not during the H1N1 pandemic: Selecting the lesser of two evils? *PLoS ONE, 8,* article e58852. doi:10.1037/t07597-000

Asmundson, G. J. G., & Taylor, S. (2005). *It's not all in your head: How worrying about your health could be making you sick—and what you can do about it.* New York: Guilford.

Asmundson, G. J. G., Taylor, S., & Cox, B. J. (2001). *Health anxiety*. New York: Wiley.

Atlani-Duault, L., Mercier, A., Rousseau, C., Guyot, P., & Moatti, J. P. (2015). Blood libel rebooted: Traditional scapegoats, online media, and the H1N1 epidemic. *Culture, Medicine and Psychiatry, 39,* 43-61. doi:10.1007/s11013-014-9410-y

Babcock, H. M., Jernigan, J. A., & Relman, D. A. (2014). The importance of influenza vaccination. *JAMA Internal Medicine, 174,* 644-645. doi:10.1001/jamainternmed.2013.11174

Bai, Y., Lin, C.-C., Lin, C.-Y., Chen, J.-Y., Chue, C.-M., & Chou, P. (2004). Survey of stress reactions among health care workers involved with the SARS outbreak. *Psychiatric Services, 55,* 1055-1057. doi:10.1176/appi.ps.55.9.1055

Bandura, A. (1986). *Social foundations of thought and action: A social cognitive theory*. Englewood Cliffs, NJ: Prentice-Hall.

Bangerter, A., Krings, F., Mouton, A., Gilles, I., Green, E. G. T., & Clémence, A. (2012). Longitudinal investigation of public trust in institutions relative to the 2009 H1N1 pandemic in Switzerland. *PLoS ONE, 7,* article e49806. doi:10.1371/journal.pone.0049806

Barlow, D. H. (2004). *Anxiety and its disorders (2nd ed.).* New York: Guilford.

Barrett, R., & Brown, P. J. (2008). Stigma in the time of influenza: Social and institutional responses to pandemic emergencies. *Journal of Infectious Diseases, 197*(Suppl 1), S34-SS37. doi:10.1086/524986

Barry, J. M. (2005). 1918 revisited: Lessons and suggestions for further inquiry. In S. L. Knobler, A. Mack, A. Mahmoud, & S. M. Lemon (Eds.),

The threat of pandemic influenza: Are we ready? (pp. 58-68). Washington, DC: National Academies Press.

Barry, J. M. (2009). Pandemics: Avoiding the mistakes of 1918. *Nature, 459*, 324-325.

Baum, N. M., Jacobson, P. D., & Goold, S. D. (2009). "Listen to the people": Public deliberation about social distancing measures in a pandemic. *American Journal of Bioethics, 9*, 4-14. doi:10.1080/15265160903197531

BBC News. (2001). HIV man guilty of infecting girlfriend, http://news.bbc.co.uk/2/hi/uk_news/scotland/1186093.stm, accessed February 4, 2019.

BBC News. (2003). China steps up SARS curbs. Retrieved from //news.bbc.co.uk/1/hi/world/asia-pacific/3002749.stm, accessed 19 Dec, 2017

Beard, K. R., Brendish, N. J., & Clark, T. W. (2018). Treatment of influenza with neuraminidase inhibitors. *Current Opinion in Infectious Diseases, 31*, 514-519. doi:10.1097/QCO.0000000000000496

Behrman, A., & Offley, W. (2013). Should influenza vaccination be mandatory for healthcare workers? *BMJ (Clinical Research Ed.), 347*, f6705-f6705. doi:10.1136/bmj.f6705

Belshe, R. (2005). The origins of pandemic influenza. *New England Journal of Medicine, 353*, 2209-2211.

Berkman, B. E. (2008). Mitigating pandemic influenza: The ethics of implementing a school closure policy. *Journal of Public Health Management and Practice, 14*, 372-378. doi:10.1097/01.PHH.0000324566.72533.0b

Betsch, C., Schmid, P., Heinemeier, D., Korn, L., Holtmann, C., & Böhm, R. (2018). Beyond confidence: Development of a measure assessing the 5C psychological antecedents of vaccination. *PLoS ONE, 13*, e0208601.

Betsch, C., Ulshöfer, C., Renkewitz, F., & Betsch, T. (2011). The influence of narrative v statistical information on perceiving vaccination risks. *Medical Decision Making, 31*, 742-753. doi:10.1177/0272989X11400419

Bird, S. E. (1996). CJ's revenge: Media, folklore, and the cultural construction of AIDS. *Critical Studies in Mass Communication, 13*, 44-58. doi:10.1080/15295039609366959

Birnie, K. A., Noel, M., Chambers, C. T., Uman, L. S., & Parker, J. A. (2018). Psychological interventions for needle-related procedural pain and distress in children and adolescents. *Cochrane Database of Systematic Reviews, 10*, CD005179.

doi:10.1002/14651858.CD005179.pub4

Birrell, J., Meares, K., Wilkinson, A., & Freeston, M. (2011). Toward a definition of intolerance of uncertainty: A review of factor analytical studies of the Intolerance of Uncertainty Scale. *Clinical Psychology Review, 31*, 1198-1208. doi:10.1016/j.cpr.2011.07.009

Bish, A., & Michie, S. (2010). Demographic and attitudinal determinants of protective behaviours during a pandemic: A review. *British Journal of Health Psychology, 15*, 797-824.

Biss, E. (2014). *On immunity: An inoculation*. Minnesota, MN: Graywolf.

Blakey, S. M., Reuman, L., Jacoby, R. J., & Abramowitz, J. S. (2015). Tracing "fearbola": Psychological predictors of anxious responding to the threat of Ebola. *Cognitive Therapy and Research, 39*, 816-825. doi:10.1007/s10608-015-9701-9

Bobevski, I., Clarke, D. M., & Meadows, G. (2016). Health anxiety and its relationship to disability and service use: Findings from a large epidemiological survey. *Psychosomatic Medicine, 78*, 13-25. doi:10.1097/PSY.0000000000000252

Boelen, P. A., & Carleton, R. N. (2012). Intolerance of uncertainty, hypochondriacal concerns, obsessive-compulsive symptoms, and worry. *Journal of Nervous and Mental Disease, 200*, 208-213. doi:10.1097/NMD.0b013e318247cb17

Böhm, R., Meier, N. W., Groß, M., Korn, L., & Betsch, C. (2018). The willingness to vaccinate increases when vaccination protects others who have low responsibility for not being vaccinated. *Journal of Behavioral Medicine*. doi:10.1007/s10865-018-9985-9

Bonneux, L., & Van Damme, W. (2010). Preventing iatrogenic pandemics of panic: Do it in a NICE way. *British Medical Journal (Clinical Research Edition), 340*, 1308.

Bora, K., Das, D., Barman, B., & Borah, P. (2018). Are internet videos useful sources of information during global public health emergencies? A case study of YouTube videos during the 2015-16 Zika virus pandemic. *Pathogens and Global Health, 112*, 320-328. doi:10.1080/20477724.2018.1507784

Born, K., Ikura, S., & Laupacis, A. (2015). The evidence, ethics and politics of mandatory health care worker vaccination. *Journal of Health Services Research & Policy, 20*, 1-3. doi:10.1177/1355819614546960

Bottesi, G., Ghisi, M., Sica, C., & Freeston, M. H. (2017). Intolerance of uncertainty, not just right experiences, and compulsive checking: Test of a moderated mediation model on a non-clinical sample. *Comprehensive Psychiatry, 73*, 111-119.

doi:10.1016/j.comppsych.2016.11.014

Bowcott, O., & Carrell, S. (2009, July 23). Swine flu website overwhelmed by demand as new cases double in a week. *The Guardian, https://www.theguardian.com/world/2009/jul/23/swine-flu-website-overwhelmed. Accessed May 3, 2018.*

Brand, J., McKay, D., Wheaton, M. G., & Abramowitz, J. S. (2013). The relationship between obsessive compulsive beliefs and symptoms, anxiety and disgust sensitivity, and Swine flu fears. *Journal of Obsessive-Compulsive and Related Disorders, 2*, 200-206. doi:10.1016/j.jocrd.2013.01.007

Brehm, J. W. (1966). *A theory of psychological reactance.* New York: Academic.

Brehm, S. S., & Brehm, J. W. (1981). *Psychological reactance: A theory of freedom and control.* New York: Academic.

Breslau, N., Peterson, E. L., & Schultz, L. R. (2008). A second look at prior trauma and the posttraumatic stress disorder effects of subsequent trauma: A prospective epidemiological study. *Archives of General Psychiatry, 65*, 431-437.

Brewer, N. T., Chapman, G. B., Gibbons, F. X., Gerrard, M., McCaul, K. D., & Weinstein, N. D. (2007). Meta-analysis of the relationship between risk perception and health behavior: The example of vaccination. *Health Psychology, 26*, 136-145. doi:10.1037/0278-6133.26.2.136

Brewin, C. R., Scragg, P., Robertson, M., Thompson, M., d'Ardenne, P., & Ehlers, A. (2008). Promoting mental health following the London bombings: A screen and treat approach. *Journal of Traumatic Stress, 21*, 3-8.

Bridges, C. B., Kuehnert, M. J., & Hall, C. B. (2003). Transmission of influenza: Implications for control in health care settings. *Clinical Infectious Diseases, 37*, 1094-1101.

Bristow, N. K. (2010). "It's as bad as anything can be": Patients, identity, and the influenza pandemic. *Public Health Reports, 125 (Suppl. 3)*, 134-144.

Bristow, N. K. (2012). *American pandemic: The lost world of the 1918 influenza epidemic.* New York: Oxford University Press.

Brooks, J. (1996). The sad and tragic life of Typhoid Mary. *Canadian Medical Association Journal, 154*, 915-916.

Bruder, M., Haffke, P., Neave, N., Nouripanah, N., & Imhoff, R. (2013). Measuring individual differences in generic beliefs in conspiracy theories across cultures: Conspiracy Mentality Questionnaire. *Frontiers in Psychology, 4*. doi:10.3389/fpsyg.2013.00225

Buhr, K., & Dugas, M. J. (2002). The Intolerance of Uncertainty Scale: Psychometric properties of the English version. *Behaviour Research and Therapy, 40*, 931-946. doi:10.1016/S0005-7967(01)00092-4

Caley, P., Philp, D. J., & McCracken, K. (2008). Quantifying social distancing arising from pandemic influenza. *Journal of the Royal Society Interface, 5*, 631-639.

Canadian Psychological Association. (2009). *Coping with concerns about the H1N1 influenza A virus and pandemics: Information for Canadians*. Ottawa: Author.

Cano-Vindel, A., Muñoz-Navarro, R., Medrano, L. A., Ruiz-Rodríguez, P., González-Blanch, C., Gómez-Castillo, M. D., . . . Santolaya, F. (2018). A computerized version of the Patient Health Questionnaire-4 as an ultra-brief screening tool to detect emotional disorders in primary care. *Journal of Affective Disorders, 234*, 247-255.

Carver, C. S., Scheier, M. F., & Segerstrom, S. C. (2010). Optimism. *Clinical Psychology Review, 30*, 879-889.

Cassady, D., Castaneda, X., Ruelas, M. R., Vostrejs, M. M., andrews, T., & Osorio, L. (2012). Pandemics and vaccines: Perceptions, reactions, and lessons learned from hard-to-reach Latinos and the H1N1 campaign. *Journal of Health Care for the Poor and Underserved, 23*, 1106-1122. doi:10.1353/hpu.2012.0086

Cauchemez, S., Ferguson, N. M., Wachtel, C., Tegnell, A., Saour, G., Duncan, B., & Nicoll, A. (2009). Closure of schools during an influenza pandemic. *Lancet Infectious Diseases, 9*, 473-481. doi:10.1186/1471-2334-14-207

Centers for Disease Control and Prevention. (2007). *Interim pre-pandemic planning guidance: Community strategy for pandemic influenza mitigation in the United States*. Washington, DC: Author.

Centers for Disease Control and Prevention. (2011). Final estimates of the 2009-10 seasonal influenza and influenza A (H1N1) 2009 monovalent vaccination coverage. Retrieved March 19, 2018, from http://www.cdc.gov/flu/professionals/vaccination/coverage_0910estimates.htm.

Centers for Disease Control and Prevention. (2018a). Guillain Barré Syndrome. https://www.cdc.gov/vaccinesafety/concerns/guillain-barre-syndrome.html, accessed February 21, 2019.

Centers for Disease Control and Prevention. (2018b). Influenza vaccination recommendations, 2017-2018, https://www.cdc.gov/vaccines/ed/flu-recs/, accessed April 10, 2018.

Chan, D. C. N., Wu, A. M. S., & Hung, E. P. W. (2010). Invulnerability and the intention to drink and drive: An application of the theory of planned behavior. *Accident Analysis and Prevention, 42*, 1549-1555. doi:10.1016/j.aap.2010.03.011

Chandavarkar, R. (1992). Plague panic and epidemic politics in India, 1896–1914. In P. Slack & T. Ranger (Eds.), *Epidemics and ideas: Essays on the historical perception of pestilence* (pp. 203-240). Cambridge: Cambridge University Press.

Channappanavar, R., & Perlman, S. (2017). Pathogenic human coronavirus infections: Causes and consequences of cytokine storm and immunopathology. *Seminars in Immunopathology, 39*, 529-539. doi:10.1007/s00281-017-0629-x

Cheng, C. (2004). To be paranoid is the standard? Panic responses to SARS out-break in the Hong Kong Special Administrative Region. *Asian Perspective, 28*, 67-98.

Cheng, C., & Cheung, M. W. (2005). Psychological responses to outbreak of severe acute respiratory syndrome: A prospective, multiple time-point study. *Journal of Personality, 73*, 261-285.

Cheng, M. C. (2005). Flu, what flu? *Lancet Infectious Diseases, 5*, 746.

Cheng, S. K., Wong, C. W., Tsang, J., & Wong, K. C. (2004). Psychological distress and negative appraisals in survivors of severe acute respiratory syndrome (SARS). *Psychological Medicine, 34*, 1187-1195.

Cichocka, A., Marchlewska, M., & Golec de Zavala, A. (2016). Does self-love or self-hate predict conspiracy beliefs? Narcissism, self-esteem, and the endorsement of conspiracy theories. *Social Psychological and Personality Science, 7*, 157-166. doi:10.1177/1948550615616170

Cichocka, A., Marchlewska, M., Golec de Zavala, A., & Olechowski, M. (2016). "They will not control us": Ingroup positivity and belief in intergroup conspiracies. *British Journal of Psychology, 107*, 556-576. doi:10.1111/bjop.12158

Clay, R. (2017). The behavioral immune system and attitudes about vaccines: Contamination aversion predicts more negative vaccine attitudes. *Social Psychological and Personality Science, 8*, 162-172. doi:10.1177/1948550616664957

Clifford, S., & Wendell, D. G. (2016). How disgust influences health purity attitudes. *Political Behavior, 38*, 155-178. doi:10.1007/s11109-015-9310-z

Cloninger, C. R. (1994). Temperament and personality. *Current Opinion in Neurobiology, 4*, 266-273.

Cohn, S. K. (2010). *Cultures of plague: Medical thinking at the end of the renaissance*. Oxford: Oxford University Press.

Collinson, S., Khan, K., & Heffernan, J. M. (2015). The effects of media reports on disease spread and important public health measurements. *PLoS ONE, 10*, e0141423. doi:10.1371/journal.pone.0141423

Cooper, K., Gregory, J. D., Walker, I., Lambe, S., & Salkovskis, P. M. (2017). Cognitive behaviour therapy for health anxiety: A systematic review and meta-analysis. *Behavioural and Cognitive Psychotherapy, 45*, 110-123. doi:10.1017/S1352465817000510

Corrard, F., Copin, C., Wollner, A., Elbez, A., Derkx, V., Bechet, S., . . . Cohen, R. (2017). Sickness behavior in feverish children is independent of the severity of fever. An observational, multicenter study. *PLoS ONE, 12*, e0171670. doi:10.1371/journal.pone.0171670

Cortes-Penfield, N. (2014). Mandatory influenza vaccination for health care workers as the new standard of care: A matter of patient safety and nonmaleficent practice. *American Journal of Public Health, 104*, 2060-2065. doi:10.2105/AJPH.2013.301514

Costa, P. T., & McCrae, R. R. (1987). Neuroticism, somatic complaints, and disease: Is the bark worse than the bite? *Journal of Personality, 55*, 299-316.

Cowling, B. J., Fung, R. O., Cheng, C. K., Fang, V. J., Chan, K. H., Seto, W. H., ... Leung, G. M. (2008). Preliminary findings of a randomized trial of nonpharmaceutical interventions to prevent influenza transmission in households. *PLoS ONE, 3*, article e2101. doi:10.1371/journal.pone.0002101

Craft, S., Ashley, S., & Maksl, A. (2017). News media literacy and conspiracy theory endorsement. *Communication and the Public, 2*, 388-401. doi:10.1177/2057047317725539

Crocker, J., Major, B., & Steele, C. (1998). Social stigma. In D. Gilbert, S. T. Fiske, & G. Lindzey (Eds.), *Handbook of social psychology* (4th ed., pp. 504-553). Boston, MA: McGraw-Hill.

Crosby, A. W. (2003). *America's forgotten pandemic: The influenza of 1918 (2nd ed.)*. Cambridge: Cambridge University Press.

Crum-Cianflone, N. F., Blair, P. J., Faix, D., Arnold, J., Echols, S., Sherman, S. S., ... Hale, B. R. (2009). Clinical and epidemiologic characteristics of an outbreak of novel H1N1 (swine origin) influenza A virus among United States military beneficiaries. *Clinical Infectious Diseases, 49*, 1801-1810. doi:10.1086/648508

Curtis, V., de Barra, M., & Aunger, R. (2011). Disgust as an adaptive system for disease avoidance behaviour. *Philosophical Transactions of the Royal Society: Series B: Biological Sciences, 366*, 389-401. doi:10.1098/rstb.2010.0117

Daley, M. F., Narwaney, K. J., Shoup, J. A., Wagner, N. M., & Glanz, J. M. (2018). Addressing parents' vaccine concerns: A randomized trial of a social media intervention. *American Journal of Preventive Medicine, 55*, 44-54. doi:10.1016/j.amepre.2018.04.010

Dantzer, R. (2009). Cytokine, sickness behavior, and depression. *Immunology and Allergy Clinics of North America, 29*, 247-264. doi:10.1016/j.iac.2009.02.002

Dantzer, R., O'Connor, J. C., Freund, G. C., Johnson, R. W., & Kelley, K. W. (2008). From inflammation to sickness and depression: When the immune system subjugates the brain. *Nature Reviews Neuroscience, 9*, 46-57.

Data-Franco, J., & Berk, M. (2013). The nocebo effect: A clinicians guide. *Australian and New Zealand Journal of Psychiatry, 47*, 617-623. doi:10.1177/0004867412464717

Davey, G. C., Hampton, J., Farrell, J., & Davidson, S. (1992). Some characteristics of worrying: Evidence for worrying and anxiety as separate constructs. *Personality and Individual Differences, 13*, 133-147. doi:10.1016/0191-8869(92)90036-O

Davis, B. M., Markel, H., Navarro, A., Wells, E., Monto, A. S., & Aiello, A. E. (2015). The effect of reactive school closure on community influenza-like illness counts in the state of Michigan during the 2009 H1N1 pandemic. *Clinical Infectious Diseases, 60*, e90-e97. doi:10.1093/cid/civ182

de Groot, J. H. B., Semin, G. R., & Smeets, M. A. M. (2014). I can see, hear, and smell your fear: Comparing olfactory and audiovisual media in fear communication. *Journal of Experimental Psychology: General, 143*, 825-834. doi:10.1037/a0033731

de Hoog, N., Stroebe, W., & de Wit, J. B. F. (2007). The impact of vulnerability to and severity of a health risk on processing and acceptance of fear-arousing communications: A meta-analysis. *Review of General Psychology, 11*, 258-285.

Debiec, J., & Olsson, A. (2017). Social fear learning: From animal models to human function. *Trends in Cognitive Sciences, 21*, 546-555. doi:10.1016/j.tics.2017.04.010

Desclaux, A., Diop, M., & Doyon, S. (2017). Fear and containment: Contact follow-up and social effects in Senegal and Guinea. In M. Hofman & S. Au (Eds.), *The politics of fear: Medecins sans Frontieres and the West African ebola epidemic* (pp. 210-234). New York: Oxford University Press.

Devine, A., Boluk, K., & Devine, F. (2017). Managing social media during a crisis: A conundrum for event managers. *Event Management, 21,* 375-389. doi:10.3727/152599517X14998876105729

Dezecache, G. (2015). Human collective reactions to threat. *WIREs Cognitive Science, 6,* 209-219. doi:10.1002/wcs.1344

Diaz, A., Soriano, J. F., & Belena, A. (2016). Perceived Vulnerability to Disease Questionnaire: Factor structure, psychometric properties and gender differences. *Personality and Individual Differences, 101,* 42-49. doi:10.1016/j.paid.2016.05.036

DiFonzo, N., & Bordia, P. (2007). *Rumor psychology: Social and organizational approaches.* Washington, DC: American Psychological Association.

Doering, B. K., & Eisma, M. C. (2016). Treatment for complicated grief: State of the science and ways forward. *Current Opinion in Psychiatry, 29,* 286-291.

Doherty, P. C. (2013). *Pandemics.* Oxford: Oxford University Press.

Dorribo, V., Lazor-Blanchet, C., Hugli, O., & Zanetti, G. (2015). Health care workers' influenza vaccination: Motivations and mandatory mask policy. *Occupational Medicine, 65,* 739-745. doi:10.1093/occmed/kqv116

Doshi, P. (2013). Influenza vaccines: Time for a rethink. *JAMA Internal Medicine, 173,* 1014-1016. doi:10.1001/jamainternmed.2013.490

Doshi, P. (2014). The importance of influenza vaccination—reply. *JAMA Internal Medicine, 174,* 645-646. doi:10.1001/jamainternmed.2013.11170

Douglas, K. M., Sutton, R. M., & Cichocka, A. (2017). The psychology of conspiracy theories. *Current Directions in Psychological Science, 26,* 538-542. doi:10.1177/0963721417718261

Douglas, K. M., Uscinski, J. E., Sutton, R. M., Cichocka, A., Nefes, T., Ang, C. S., & Deravi, F. (2019). Understanding conspiracy theories. *Political Psychology, 40,* 3-35. doi:10.1111/pops.12568

Douglas, P. K., Douglas, D. B., Harrigan, D. C., & Douglas, K. M. (2009). Preparing for pandemic influenza and its aftermath: Mental health issues considered. *International Journal of Emergency Mental Health, 11,* 137-144.

Dugas, M. J., & Robichaud, M. (2007). *Cognitive-behavioral treatment for generalized anxiety disorder: From science to practice.* New York: Routledge.

Duncan, L. A., & Schaller, M. (2009). Prejudicial attitudes toward older adults may be exaggerated when people feel vulnerable to infectious disease: Evidence and implications. *Analyses of Social Issues and Public Policy, 9*, 97-115. doi:j.1530-2415.2009.01188.x

Duncan, L. A., Schaller, M., & Park, J. H. (2009). Perceived vulnerability to disease: Development and validation of a 15-item self-report instrument. *Personality and Individual Differences, 47*, 541-546. doi:10.1016/j.paid.2009.05.001

Ecker, W., Kupfer, J., & Gönner, S. (2014). Incompleteness and harm avoidance in OCD, anxiety and depressive disorders, and non-clinical controls. *Journal of Obsessive-Compulsive and Related Disorders, 3*, 46-51. doi:10.1016/j.jocrd.2013.12.001

EHS Today. (2000). Restaurant corporation first to mandate hepatitis vaccine, https://www.ehstoday.com/news/ehs_imp_32892, accessed February 8, 2019.

Eichelberger, L. (2007). SARS and New York's Chinatown: The politics of risk and blame during an epidemic of fear. *Social Science & Medicine, 65*, 1284-1295.

Eichner, M., Schwehm, M., Duerr, H.-P., Witschi, M., Koch, D., Brockmann, S. O., & Vidondo, B. (2009). Antiviral prophylaxis during pandemic influenza may increase drug resistance. *BMC Infectious Diseases, 9*, article 4. doi:10.1186/1471-2334-9-4

Eilenberg, T., Frostholm, L., Schroder, A., Jensen, J. S., & Fink, P. (2015). Long-term consequences of severe health anxiety on sick leave in treated and untreated patients: Analysis alongside a randomised controlled trial. *Journal of Anxiety Disorders, 32*, 95-102. doi:10.1016/j.janxdis.2015.04.001

Epstein, G. A. (2003). Amid SARS epidemic, China panics over pets. *Baltimore Sun*, https://www.baltimoresun.com/bal-te.china06may06-story.html, accessed March 26, 2019.

Erasmus, V., Daha, T. J., Brug, H., Richardus, J. H., Behrendt, M. D., Vos, M. C., & van Beeck, E. F. (2010). Systematic review of studies on compliance with hand hygiene guidelines in hospital care. *Infection Control & Hospital Epidemiology, 31*, 283-294.

Ernst, E. (2010). Homeopathy: What does the "best" evidence tell us? *Medical Journal of Australia, 192*, 458-460.

Evans, R. J. (1992). Epidemics and revolutions: Cholera in nineteenth-century Europe. In P. Slack & T. Ranger (Eds.), *Epidemics and ideas: Essays on the historical perception of pestilence* (pp. 149-174). Cambridge: Cambridge University Press.

Faulkner, J., Schaller, M., Park, J. H., & Duncan, L. A. (2004). Evolved disease-avoidance mechanisms and contemporary xenophobic attitudes. *Group Processes and Intergroup Behavior, 7*, 333-353. doi:10.1177/1368430204046142

Fergus, T. A. (2015). Anxiety sensitivity and intolerance of uncertainty as potential risk factors for cyberchondria: A replication and extension examining dimensions of each construct. *Journal of Affective Disorders, 184*, 305-309. doi:10.1016/j.jad.2015.06.017

Fergus, T. A., Bardeen, J. R., & Orcutt, H. K. (2015). Examining the specific facets of distress tolerance that are relevant to health anxiety. *Journal of Cognitive Psychotherapy, 29*, 32-44. doi:10.1891/0889-8391.29.1.32

Ferguson, E. (2000). Hypochondriacal concerns and the five-factor model of personality. *Journal of Personality, 68*, 705-724.

Fine, P., Eames, K., & Heymann, D. L. (2011). "Herd immunity": A rough guide. *Clinical Infectious Diseases, 52*, 911-916. doi:10.1093/cid/cir007

Finkelstein, S., Prakash, S., Nigmatulina, K., Klaiman, T., & Larson, R. (2010). Pandemic influenza: Non-pharmaceutical interventions and behavioral changes that may save lives. *International Journal of Health Management and Information, 1*, 1-18.

Ford, E. W., Boyer, B. T., Menachemi, N., & Huerta, T. R. (2014). Increasing hand washing compliance with a simple visual cue. *American Journal of Public Health, 104*, 1851-1856.

Fraser, C., Donnelly, C. A., Cauchemez, S., Hanage, W. P., Van Kerkhove, M. D., Hollingsworth, T. D., . . . Roth, C. (2009). Pandemic potential of a strain of influenza A (H1N1): Early findings. *Science, 324*, 1557-1561. doi:10.1126/science.1176062

Frederick, J., Brown, A. C., Cummings, D. A., Gaydos, C. A., Gibert, C. L., Gorse, G. J., . . . Simberkoff, M. S. (2018). Protecting healthcare personnel in outpatient settings: The influence of mandatory versus nonmandatory influenza vaccination policies on workplace absenteeism during multiple respiratory virus seasons. *Infection Control and Hospital Epidemiology, 39*, 452-461. doi:10.1017/ice.2018.9

Frost, K., Frank, E., & Maibach, E. (1997). Relative risk in the news media: A quantification of misrepresentation. *American Journal of Public Health, 87*, 842-845.

Frost, R. O., & Steketee, G. (2002). *Cognitive approaches to obsessions and compulsions: Theory, assessment, and treatment.* Oxford: Elsevier.

Furuya-Kanamori, L., Cox, M., Milinovich, G. J., Magalhaes, R. J. S., Mackay, I. M., & Yakob, L. (2016). Heterogeneous and dynamic prevalence of asymptomatic influenza virus infections. *Emerging Infectious Diseases, 22*, 1052-1056. doi:10.3201/eid2206.151080

Galliford, N., & Furnham, A. (2017). Individual difference factors and beliefs in medical and political conspiracy theories. *Scandinavian Journal of Psychology, 58*, 422-428. doi:10.1111/sjop.12382

Galvani, A. P., & May, R. M. (2005). Dimensions of superspreading. *Nature, 438*, 293-295.

Gardner, P. J., & Moallef, P. (2015). Psychological impact on SARS survivors: Critical review of the English language literature. *Canadian Psychology, 56*, 123-135.

Gautreau, C. M., Sherry, S. B., Sherry, D. L., Birnie, K. A., Mackinnon, S. P., & Stewart, S. H. (2015). Does catastrophizing of bodily sensations maintain health-related anxiety? A 14-day daily diary study with longitudinal follow-up. *Behavioural and Cognitive Psychotherapy, 43*, 502-512. doi:10.1017/S1352465814000150

Gentes, E. L., & Ruscio, A. M. (2011). A meta-analysis of the relation of intolerance of uncertainty to symptoms of generalized anxiety disorder, major depressive disorder, and obsessive–compulsive disorder. *Clinical Psychology Review, 31*, 923-933. doi:10.1016/j.cpr.2011.05.001

Georges-Courbot, M. C., Leroy, E., & Zeller, H. (2002). Ebola: Un virus endemique en Afrique centrale? *Medecine Tropicale: Revue Du Corps De Sante Colonial, 62*, 295-300.

Getz, W. M., Carlson, C., Dougherty, E., Porco Francis, Travis C., & Salter, R. (2016). An agent-based model of school closing in under-vacccinated communities during measles outbreaks. *Agent-Directed Simulation Symposium, 2016.*

Gibbons, F. X., Gerrard, M., & Pomery, E. A. (2004). Risk and reactance. In R. A. Wright, J. Greenberg, & S. S. Brehm (Eds.), *Motivational analyses of social behavior* (pp. 149-166). Mahwah, NJ: Erlbaum.

Gilles, I., Bangerter, A., Clémence, A., Green, E. G. T., Krings, F., Mouton, A., . . . Wagner-Egger, P. (2013). Collective symbolic coping with disease threat and othering: A case study of avian influenza. *British Journal of Social Psychology, 52*, 83-102.

Gilles, I., Bangerter, A., Clémence, A., Green, E. G. T., Krings, F., Staerklé, C., & Wagner-Egger, P. (2011). Trust in medical organizations predicts pandemic (H1N1) 2009 vaccination behavior and perceived efficacy of protection measures in the Swiss public. *European Journal of Epidemiology, 26*, 203-210.

Glanz, J. M., Wagner, N. M., Narwaney, K. J., Kraus, C. R., Shoup, J. A., Xu, S., . . . Daley, M. F. (2017). Web-based social media intervention to increase vaccine acceptance: A randomized controlled trial. *Pediatrics, 140*. doi:10.1542/peds.2017-1117

Glaser, R., & Kiecolt-Glaser, J. K. (2005). Stress-induced immune dysfunction: Implications for health. *Nature Reviews Immunology, 5*, 243-251. doi:10.1038/nri1571

Godinho, C. A., Yardley, L., Marcu, A., Mowbray, F., Beard, E., & Michie, S. (2016). Increasing the intent to receive a pandemic influenza vaccination: Testing the impact of theory-based messages. *Preventive Medicine, 89*, 104-111.

Godlee, F., Smith, J., & Marcovitch, H. (2011). Wakefield's article linking MMR vaccine and autism was fraudulent. *British Medical Journal, 342*, c7452.

Goetz, A. R., Lee, H., Cougle, J. R., & Turkel, J. E. (2013). Disgust propensity and sensitivity: Differential relationships with obsessive–compulsive symptoms and behavioral approach task performance. *Journal of Obsessive Compulsive and Related Disorders, 2*, 412-419.

Goffman, E. (1963). *Stigma: Notes on the management of spoiled identity*. New York: Simon and Schuster.

Goldenberg, J. L., & Arndt, J. (2008). The implications of death for health: A terror management health model for behavioral health promotion. *Psychological Review, 115*, 1032-1053.

Goodwin, R., Gaines, S. O., Myers, L., & Neto, F. (2009). Initial psychological reactions to swine flu. *International Journal of Behavioral Medicine, 18*, 88-92.

Gouglas, D., Le, T. T., Henderson, K., Kaloudis, A., Danielsen, T., Hammersland, N. C., . . . Rottingen, J.-A. (2018). Estimating the cost of vaccine developent against epidemic infectious diseases: A cost minimisation study. *Lancet Global Health*. doi:10.1016/S2214-109X(18)30346-2

Goumon, S., & Špinka, M. (2016). Emotional contagion of distress in young pigs is potentiated by previous exposure to the same stressor. *Animal Cognition, 19*, 501-511. doi:10.1007/s10071-015-0950-5

Grant, L., Hausman, B. L., Cashion, M., Lucchesi, N., Patel, K., & Roberts, J. (2015). Vaccination persuasion online: A qualitative study of two provaccine and two vaccine-skeptical websites. *Journal of Medical Internet Research, 17*. doi:10.2196/jmir.4153

Graves, C. (1969). *Invasion by virus: Can it happen again?* London: Icon Books.

Green, E. G., Krings, F., Staerklé, C., Bangerter, A., Clémence, A., Wagner-Egger, P., & Bornand, T. (2010). Keeping the vermin out: Perceived disease threat and ideological orientations as predictors of exclusionary immigration attitudes. *Journal of Community Applied Social Psychology, 20*, 299-316.

Green, J. S., & Teachman, B. A. (2013). Predictive validity of explicit and implicit threat overestimation in contamination fear. *Journal of Obsessive-Compulsive and Related Disorders, 2*, 1-8.

Grimaud, J., & Legagneur, F. (2011). Community beliefs and fears during a cholera outbreak in Haiti. *Intervention: International Journal of Mental Health, Psychosocial Work & Counselling in Areas of Armed Conflict, 9*, 26-34. doi:dx.doi.org/10.1097/WTF.0b013e3283453ef2

Gruben, V., Siemieniuk, R. A., & McGeer, A. (2014). Health care workers, mandatory influenza vaccination policies and the law. *Canadian Medical Association Journal, 186*, 1076-1080. doi:10.1503/cmaj.140035

Gruenberg, D. A., & Shaker, M. S. (2011). An update on influenza vaccination in patients with egg allergy. *Current Opinion in Pediatrics, 23*, 566-572.

Grzesiak-Feldman, M. (2013). The effect of high-anxiety situations on conspiracy thinking. *Current Psychology, 32*, 100-118. doi:10.1007/s12144-013-9165-6

Gump, B. B., & Kulik, J. A. (1997). Stress, affiliation, and emotional contagion. *Journal of Personality and Social Psychology, 72*, 305-319.

Haase, N., Betsch, C., & Renkewitz, F. (2015). Source credibility and the biasing effect of narrative information on the perception of vaccination risks. *Journal of Health Communication, 20*, 920-929. doi:10.1080/10810730.2015.1018605

Hagger, M. S., Koch, S., Chatzisarantis, N. L. D., & Orbell, S. (2017). The common sense model of self-regulation: Meta-analysis and test of a process model. *Psychological Bulletin, 143*, 1117-1154. doi:10.1037/bul0000118

Hakim, H., Provencher, T., Chambers, C. T., Driedger, S. M., Dube, E., Gavaruzzi, T., . . . Witteman, H. O. (2019). Interventions to help people understand community immunity: A systematic review. *Vaccine, 37*, 235-247. doi:10.1016/j.vaccine.2018.11.016

Hall, M. G., Sheeran, P., Noar, S. M., Ribisl, K. M., Boynton, M. H., & Brewer, N. T. (2017). A brief measure of reactance to health warnings. *Journal of Behavioral Medicine, 40*, 520-529. doi:10.1007/s10865-016-9821-z

Hammond, C., Holmes, D., & Mercier, M. (2016). Breeding new forms of life: A critical reflection on extreme variances of bareback sex. *Nursing Inquiry, 23*, 267-277. doi:10.1111/nin.12139

Hatfield, E., Cacioppo, J. T., & Rapson, R. L. (1994). *Emotional contagion.* Cambridge, England: Cambridge University Press.

Hatfield, E., Carpenter, M., & Rapson, R. L. (2014). Emotional contagion as a precursor to collective emotions. In C. von Scheve & M. Salmela (Eds.), *Collective emotions: Perspectives from psychology, philosophy, and sociology.* (pp. 108-122). New York: Oxford University Press.

Heagerty, J. J. (1919). Influenza and vaccination. *Canadian Medical Association Journal, 9*, 226-228.

Hedman, E., Lekander, M., Karshikoff, B., Ljótsson, B., Axelsson, E., & Axelsson, J. (2016). Health anxiety in a disease-avoidance framework: Investigation of anxiety, disgust and disease perception in response to sickness cues. *Journal of Abnormal Psychology, 125*, 868-878.

Heller, J. (2015). Rumors and realities: Making sense of HIV/AIDS conspiracy narratives and contemporary legends. *American Journal of Public Health, 105*, e43-e50.

Herrera-Valdez, M. A., Cruz-Aponte, M., & Castillo-Chavez, C. (2011). Multiple outbreaks for the same pandemic: Local transportation and social distancing explain the different "waves" of A-H1N1pdm cases observed in México during 2009. *Mathematical Biosciences and Engineering, 8*, 21-48. doi:10.3934/mbe.2011.8.21

Hill, P. L., Duggan, P. M., & Lapsley, D. K. (2012). Subjective invulnerability, risk behavior, and adjustment in early adolescence. *Journal of Early Adolescence, 32*, 489-501. doi:10.1177/0272431611400304

Hoegh, A., Ferreira, M. A. R., & Leman, S. (2016). Spatiotemporal model fusion: Multiscale modelling of civil unrest. *Journal of the Royal Statistical Society: Series C (Applied Statistics), 65*, 529-545. doi:10.1111/rssc.12138

Holmes, E. A. F., Hughes, D. A., & Morrison, V. L. (2014). Predicting adherence to medications using health psychology theories: A systematic review of 20 years of empirical research. *Value in Health, 17*, 863-876. doi:10.1016/j.jval.2014.08.2671

Hong, X., Currier, G. W., Zhao, X., Jiang, Y., Zhou, W., & Wei, J. (2009). Posttraumatic stress disorder in convalescent severe acute respiratory syndrome patients: A 4-year follow-up study. *General Hospital Psychiatry, 31*, 546-554.

Honigsbaum, M. (2005, March 20). On a wing and a prayer. *The Guardian, https://www.theguardian.com/world/2005/mar/20/birdflu.features, accessed April 12, 2018.*

Honigsbaum, M. (2009). *Living with Enza: The forgotten story of Britain and the great flu pandemic of 1918.* London: Macmillan.

Honigsbaum, M. (2014). *A history of the great influenza pandemics.* London: Tauris.

Hornsey, M. J., & Fielding, K. S. (2017). Attitude roots and Jiu Jitsu persuasion: Understanding and overcoming the motivated rejection of science. *American Psychologist, 72,* 459-473.

Hornsey, M. J., Harris, E. A., & Fielding, K. S. (2018). The psychological roots of anti-vaccination attitudes: A 24-nation investigation. *Health Psychology, 37,* 307-315.

House, T., Baguelin, M., Van Hoek, A. J., White, P. J., Sadique, Z., Eames, K., . . . Keeling, M. J. (2011). Modelling the impact of local reactive school closures on critical care provision during an influenza pandemic. *Proceedings of the Royal Society B: Biological Sciences, 278,* 2753-2760. doi:10.1098/rspb.2010.2688

Huang, W.-L., Chen, T.-T., Chen, I. M., Chang, L.-R., Lin, Y.-H., Liao, S.-C., & Gau, S. S.-F. (2016). Harm avoidance and persistence are associated with somatoform disorder psychopathology: A study in Taiwan. *Journal of Affective Disorders, 196,* 83-86. doi:10.1016/j.jad.2016.02.009

Huang, Y., Xu, K., Ren, D. F., Ai, J., Ji, H., Ge, A. H., . . . Wang, H. (2014). Probable longer incubation period for human infection with avian influenza A(H7N9) virus in Jiangsu Province, China, 2013. *Epidemiology and Infection, 142,* 2647-2653. doi:10.1017/S0950268814000272

Imhoff, R., & Lamberty, P. (2018). How paranoid are conspiracy believers? Toward a more fine-grained understanding of the connect and disconnect between paranoia and belief in conspiracy theories. *European Journal of Social Psychology.* doi:10.1002/ejsp.2494

Inter-Agency Standing Committee. (2007). *IASC guidelines on mental health and psychosocial support in emergency settings.* Geneva, Switzerland: Author.

Irwin, M. R., & Slavich, G. M. (2017). Psychoneuroimmunology. In J. T. Cacioppo, L. G. Tassinary, & G. G. Berntson (Eds.), *Handbook of psychophysiology., 4th ed.* (pp. 377-397). New York: Cambridge University Press.

Jacobs, A., Perpetua, S., Sreeharsha, V., McNeil, D. G., & Tavernise, S. (2016). Conspiracy theories about Zika spread through Brazil with the virus. *New York Times, 165*(57145), A6-A6.

Janssen, E., van Osch, L., de Vries, H., & Lechner, L. (2013). The influence of narrative risk communication on feelings of cancer risk. *British Journal of Health Psychology, 18*, 407-419. doi:10.1111/j.2044-8287.2012.02098.x

Jefferson, A., Bortolotti, L., & Kuzmanovic, B. (2017). What is unrealistic optimism? *Consciousness and Cognition, 50*, 3-11. doi:10.1016/j.concog.2016.10.005

Jefferson, T., Del Mar, C. B., Dooley, L., Ferroni, E., Al-Ansary, L. A., Bawazeer, G. A., . . . Conly, J. M. (2011). Physical interventions to interrupt or reduce the spread of respiratory viruses. *Cochrane Database of Systematic Reviews, 7*, article number CD006207.

Ji, L.-J., Zhang, Z., Usborne, E., & Guan, Y. (2004). Optimism across cultures: In response to the severe acute respiratory syndrome outbreak. *Asian Journal of Social Psychology, 7*, 25-34. doi:10.1111/j.1467-839X.2004.00132.x

Joffe, H. (1999). *Risk and the "other"*. Cambridge: Cambridge University Press.

Johnson, N. (2006). *Britain and the 1918-19 influenza pandemic*. New York: Routledge.

Johnson, N., & Mueller, J. (2002). Updating the accounts: Global mortality of the 1918–1920 "Spanish" influenza pandemic. *Bulletin of the History of Medicine, 76*, 105-115.

Jolley, D., & Douglas, K. M. (2014). The effects of anti-vaccine conspiracy theories on vaccination intentions. *PLoS ONE, 9*, e89177. doi:10.1371/journal.pone.0089177

Jolley, D., & Douglas, K. M. (2017). Prevention is better than cure: Addressing anti-vaccine conspiracy theories. *Journal of Applied Social Psychology, 47*, 459-469. doi:10.1111/jasp.12453

Jones, J. H., & Salathe, M. (2009). Early assessment of anxiety and behavioural response to novel swine-origin Influenza A(H1N1). *PLoS ONE, 4*, article e8032. doi:10.1371/journal.pone.0008032

Jones-Berry, S. (2018). Compulsory flu jab for staff: Is it a moral duty, or a morale wrecker? *Nursing Standard, 33*, 8-10. doi:10.7748/ns.33.3.8.s5

Judah, G., Donachie, P., Cobb, E., Schmidt, W., Holland, M., & Curtis, V. (2010). Dirty hands: Bacteria of faecal origin on commuters' hands. *Epidemiology and Infection, 138*, 409-414.

Kam, C., & Meyer, J. P. (2012). Do optimism and pessimism have different relationships with personality dimensions? A re-examination. *Personality and Individual Differences, 52*, 123-127. doi:10.1016/j.paid.2011.09.011

Kanadiya, M. K., & Sallar, A. M. (2011). Preventive behaviors, beliefs, and anxieties in relation to the swine flu outbreak among college students aged 18–24 years. *Journal of Public Health, 19*, 139-145. doi:10.1007/s10389-010-0373-3

Karademas, E. C., Bati, A., Karkania, V., Georgiou, V., & Sofokleous, S. (2013). The association between pandemic influenza A (H1N1) public perceptions and reactions: A prospective study. *Journal of Health Psychology, 18*, 419-428.

Kawaguchi, R., Miyazono, M., Noda, T., Takayama, Y., Sasai, Y., & Iso, H. (2009). Influenza (H1N1) 2009 outbreak and school closure, Osaka Prefecture, Japan. *Emerging Infectious Diseases, 15*, 1685-1685. doi:10.3201/eid1510.091029

Keil, U., Schönhöfer, P., & Spelsberg, A. (2011). The invention of the swine-flu pandemic. *European Journal of Epidemiology, 26*, 187-190. doi:10.1007/s10654-011-9573-6

Kelland, K. (2017). Proliferation of bird flu outbreaks raises risk of human pandemic. *Scientific American,* https://www.scientificamerican.com/article/proliferation-of-bird-flu-outbreaks-raises-risk-of-human-pandemic1/, accessed September 14, 2018.

Kennedy, W. P. (1961). The nocebo reaction. *Medical World, 95*, 203-205.

Kiecolt-Glaser, J. K. (2009). Psychoneuroimmunology: Psychology's gateway to the biomedical future. *Perspectives on Psychological Science, 4*, 367-369.

Kilbourne, E. D. (1977). Influenza pandemics in perspective. *Journal of the American Medical Association, 237*, 1225-1228.

Kilgo, D. K., Yoo, J., & Johnson, T. J. (2018). Spreading Ebola panic: Newspaper and social media coverage of the 2014 Ebola health crisis. *Health Communication*, 1-7. doi:10.1080/10410236.2018.1437524

Kim, H. K., & Niederdeppe, J. (2013). Exploring optimistic bias and the integrative model of behavioral prediction in the context of a campus influenza outbreak. *Journal of Health Communication, 18*, 206-222. doi:10.1080/10810730.2012.688247

Kim, M., & Choi, Y. (2017). Risk communication: The roles of message appeal and coping style. *Social Behavior & Personality, 45*, 773-784. doi:10.2224/sbp.6327

Kleiman, E. M., Chiara, A. M., Liu, R. T., Jager-Hyman, S. G., Choi, J. Y., & Alloy, L. B. (2017). Optimism and well-being: A prospective multi-method and multi-dimensional examination of optimism as a resilience factor following the occurrence of stressful life events. *Cognition and Emotion, 31*, 269-283. doi:10.1080/02699931.2015.1108284

Klemm, C., Das, E., & Hartmann, T. (2016). Swine flu and hype: A systematic review of media dramatization of the H1N1 influenza pandemic. *Journal of Risk Research, 19*, 1-20.

Knowler, P., Barrett, M., & Watson, D. A. (2018). Attitudes of healthcare workers to influenza vaccination. *Infection, Disease & Health, 23*, 156-162. doi:10.1016/j.idh.2018.03.003

Koh, D., Lim, M. K., Chia, S. E., Ko, S. M., Qian, F., Ng, V., . . . Fones, C. (2005). Risk perception and impact of severe acute respiratory syndrome (SARS) on work and personal lives of healthcare workers in Singapore: What can we learn? *Medical Care, 43*, 676-682. doi:10.1097/01.mlr.0000167181.36730.cc

Kring, A. M., & Sloan, D. M. (2010). *Emotion regulation and psychopathology: A transdiagnostic approach to etiology and treatment*. New York: Guilford.

Krug, R. M. (2003). The potential use of influenza virus as an agent for bioterrorism. *Antiviral Research, 57*, 147-150.

Kuntz, J. L., Firemark, A., Schneider, J., Henninger, M., Bok, K., & Naleway, A. (2019). Development of an intervention to reduce pain and prevent syncope related to adolescent vaccination. *The Permanente Journal, 23*. doi:10.7812/TPP/17-136

Lahrach, Y., & Furnham, A. (2017). Are modern health worries associated with medical conspiracy theories? *Journal of Psychosomatic Research, 99*, 89-94. doi:10.1016/j.jpsychores.2017.06.004

Lambert, J. (2019). Measles cases mount in Pacific Northwest outbreak. *https://www.npr.org/sections/health-shots/2019/02/08/692665531/measles-cases-mount-in-pacific-northwest-outbreak*, accessed Februrary 21, 2019.

Lantian, A., Muller, D., Nurra, C., & Douglas, K. M. (2017). "I know things they don't know!": The role of need for uniqueness in belief in conspiracy theories. *Social Psychology, 48*, 160-173. doi:10.1027/1864-9335/a000306

Lau, J. T. F., Kim, J. H., Tsui, H. Y., & Griffiths, S. (2008). Perceptions related to bird-to-human avian influenza, influenza vaccination, and use of face mask. *Infection, 36*, 434-443. doi:10.1007/s15010-008-7277-y

Lau, M. S. Y., Dalziel, B. D., Funk, S., McClelland, A., Tiffany, A., Riley, S., . . . Grenfell, B. T. (2017). Spatial and temporal dynamics of superspreading events in the 2014-2015 West Africa Ebola epidemic. *Proceedings of the National Academy of Sciences, 114*, 2337-2342. doi:10.1073/pnas.1614595114

Lauriola, M., Mosca, O., Trentini, C., Foschi, R., Tambelli, R., & Carleton, R. N. (2018). The Intolerance and Uncertainty Inventory: Validity and comparison of scoring methods to assess individuals screening positive for anxiety and depression. *Frontiers in Psychology, 9*, article 388, doi.org/310.3389/fpsyg.2018.00388.

Laver, G., & Webster, R. G. (2001). Introduction. *Philosophical Transactions of the Royal Society B: Biological Sciences, 356*, 1813-1815.

Lederberg, J., Shope, R. E., & Oakes, S. C. (1992). *Emerging infection: Microbial threats to health in the United States.* Washington, DC: National Academy Press.

Lee, J. D. (2014). *An epidemic of rumors: How stories shape our perception of disease.* Boulder, CO: University Press of Colorado.

Leibu, R., & Maslow, J. (2015). Effectiveness and acceptance of a health care-based mandatory vaccination program. *Journal of Occupational and Environmental Medicine, 57*, 58-61. doi:10.1097/JOM.0000000000000294

Leventhal, H., Phillips, L. A., & Burns, E. (2016). The common-sense model of self-regulation (CSM): A dynamic framework for understanding illness self-management. *Journal of Behavioral Medicine, 39*, 935-946.

Levi, J., Segal, L. M., St. Laurent, R., & Lieberman, D. A. (2010). Fighting flu fatigue. Retrieved April 7, 2019 from healthyamericans.org/assets/files/TFAH2010FluBriefFINAL.pdf.

Lewandowsky, S., Oberauer, K., & Gignac, G. E. (2013). NASA faked the moon landing—therefore, (climate) science is a hoax: An anatomy of the motivated rejection of science. *Psychological Science, 24*, 622-633. doi:10.1177/0956797612457686

Li, C., Hatta, M., Nidom, C. A., Muramoto, Y., Watanabe, S., Neumann, G., & Kawaoko, Y. (2010). Reassortment between avian H5N1 and human H3N2 influenza viruses creates hybrid viruses with substantial virulence. *Proceedings of the National Academy of Sciences, 107*, 4687-4692. doi:10.1073/pnas.0912807107

Li, T., Feng, J., Qing, P., Fan, X., Liu, W., Li, M., & Wang, M. (2014). Attitudes, practices and information needs regarding novel influenza A (H7N9) among employees of food production and operation in Guangzhou, Southern China: A cross-sectional study. *BMC Infectious Disease, 14*, article 4, doi: 10.1186/1471-2334-1114-1184.

Liao, Q., Cowling, B. J., Lam, W. T., & Fielding, R. (2011). Changing perception of avian influenza risk, Hong Kong, 2006–2010. *Emerging Infectious Diseases, 17*, 2379-2380.

Liu, Q., Zhou, Y., & Yang, Z. (2016). The cytokine storm of severe influenza and development of immunomodulatory therapy. *Cellular and Molecular Immunology, 13*, 3-10. doi:10.1038/cmi.2015.74

Lloyd-Smith, J. O., Schreiber, S. J., Kopp, P. E., & Getz, W. M. (2005). Superspreading and the effect of individual variation on disease emergence. *Nature, 438*, 355-359.

Logan, J., Nederhoff, D., Koch, B., Griffith, B., Wolfson, J., Awan, F. A., & Basta, N. E. (2018). "What have you HEARD about the HERD?" Does education about local influenza vaccination coverage and herd immunity affect willingness to vaccinate? *Vaccine, 36*, 4118-4125. doi:10.1016/j.vaccine.2018.05.037

Lowrie, M. (2019). McGill science group takes aim at pharmacies for selling "quack" flu remedy. *National Post*, https://nationalpost.com/pmn/news-pmn/canada-news-pmn/mcgill-science-group-takes-aim-at-pharmacies-for-selling-quack-flu-remedy, accessed January 19, 2019.

Lu, Y.-C., Shu, B.-C., Chang, Y.-Y., & Lung, F.-W. (2006). The mental health of hospital workers dealing with severe acute respiratory syndrome. *Psychotherapy and Psychosomatics, 75*, 370-375.

Ludvik, D., Boschen, M. J., & Neumann, D. L. (2015). Effective behavioural strategies for reducing disgust in contamination-related OCD: A review. *Clinical Psychology Review, 42*, 116-129.

Lukich, N., Kekewich, M., & Roth, V. (2018). Should influenza vaccination be mandatory for healthcare workers? *Healthcare Management Forum, 31*, 214-217. doi:10.1177/0840470418794209

Lutz, B. D., Bronze, M. S., & Greenfield, R. A. (2003). Influenza virus: Natural disease and bioterrorism threat. *Journal of the Oklahoma State Medical Association, 96*, 27-28.

Magallares, A., Fuster-Ruiz De Apodaca, M. J., & Morales, J. F. (2017). Psychometric properties and criterion validity of the Perceived Vulnerability to Disease Scale (PVD) in the Spanish population. *Revista de Psicología Social, 32*, 164-195. doi:10.1080/02134748.2016.1248025

Maharaj, S., & Kleczkowski, A. (2012). Controlling epidemic spread by social distancing: Do it well or not at all. *BMC Public Health, 12*, 679. doi:610.1186/1471-2458-1112-1679.

Makhanova, A., Miller, S. L., & Maner, J. K. (2015). Germs and the outgroup: Chronic and situational disease concerns affect intergroup categorization. *Evolutionary Behavioral Sciences, 9*, 8-19.

Makridakis, S., & Moleskis, A. (2015). The costs and benefits of positive illusions. *Frontiers in Psychology, 6*. doi:10.3389/fpsyg.2015.00859

Maltezou, H. C., Theodoridou, K., Ledda, C., Rapisarda, V., & Theodoridou, M. (2018). Vaccination of healthcare workers: Is mandatory vaccination needed? *Expert Review of Vaccines*. doi:10.1080/14760584.2019.1552141

Mamelund, S.-E. (2018). 1918 pandemic morbidity: The first wave hits the poor, the second wave hits the rich. *Influenza and Other Respiratory Viruses, 12*, 307-313. doi:10.1111/irv.12541

Marchlewska, M., Cichocka, A., & Kossowska, M. (2018). Addicted to answers: Need for cognitive closure and the endorsement of conspiracy beliefs. *European Journal of Social Psychology, 48*, 109-117. doi:10.1002/ejsp.2308

Mathes, B. M., Norr, A. M., Allan, N. P., Albanese, B. J., & Schmidt, N. B. (2018). Cyberchondria: Overlap with health anxiety and unique relations with impairment, quality of life, and service utilization. *Psychiatry Research, 261*, 204-211. doi:10.1016/j.psychres.2018.01.002

Mathie, R. T., Frye, J., & Fisher, P. (2015). Homeopathic Oscilloconninum for preventing and treating influenza and influenza-like illness. *Cochdrane Database of Systematic Reviews, 1*, CD001957, 001910.001002/14651858.CD14001957.pub14651856.

Maunder, R. G., Lancee, W. J., Balderson, K. E., Bennett, J. P., Borgundvaag, B., Evans, S., . . . Wasylenki, D. A. (2006). Long-term psychological and occupational effects of providing hospital healthcare during SARS outbreak. *Emerging Infectious Diseases, 12*, 1924-1932.

Mauro, C., Reynolds, C. F., Maercker, A., Skritskaya, N., Simon, N., Zisook, S., . . . Shear, M. K. (2018). Prolonged grief disorder: Clinical utility of ICD-11 diagnostic guidelines. *Psychological Medicine*.

doi:10.1017/S0033291718001563

McDonnell, W. M., Nelson, D. S., & Schunk, J. E. (2012). Should we fear "flu fear" itself? Effects of H1N1 influenza fear on ED use. *American Journal of Emergency Medicine, 30*, 275-282. doi:10.1016/j.ajem.2010.11.027

McEvoy, P. M., & Mahoney, A. E. J. (2013). Intolerance of uncertainty and negative metacognitive beliefs as transdiagnostic mediators of repetitive negative thinking in a clinical sample with anxiety disorders. *Journal of Anxiety Disorders, 27*, 216-224. doi:10.1016/j.janxdis.2013.01.006

McMurtry, C. M., Taddio, A., Noel, M., Antony, M. M., Chambers, C. T., Asmundson, G. J. G., . . . Scott, J. (2016). Exposure-based interventions for the management of individuals with high levels of needle fear across the lifespan: A clinical practice guideline and call for further research. *Cognitive Behaviour Therapy, 45*, 217-235. doi:10.1080/16506073.2016.1157204

Megiddo, I., Drabik, D., Bedford, T., Morton, A., Wesseler, J., & Laxminarayan, R. (2019). Investing in antibiotics to alleviate future catastrophic outcomes: What is the value of having an effective antibiotic to mitigate pandemic influenza? *Health Economics*, doi.org/10.1002/hec.3867.

Melli, G., Chiorri, C., Carraresi, C., Stopani, E., & Bulli, F. (2015). The two dimensions of contamination fear in obsessive-compulsive disorder: Harm avoidance and disgust avoidance. *Journal of Obsessive-Compulsive and Related Disorders, 6*, 124-131. doi:10.1016/j.jocrd.2015.07.001

Meuret, A. E., Simon, E., Bhaskara, L., & Ritz, T. (2017). Ultra-brief behavioral skills trainings for blood injection injury phobia. *Depression and Anxiety, 34*, 1096-1105. doi:10.1002/da.22616

Miller, S. M. (1987). Monitoring and blunting: Validation of a questionnaire to assess styles of information seeking under threat. *Journal of Personality and Social Psychology, 52*, 345-353.

Miller, S. M. (1988). The interacting effects of coping styles and situational variables in gynecologic settings: Implications for research and treatment. *Journal of Psychosomatic Obstetrics & Gynecology, 9*, 23-34. doi:10.3109/01674828809030946

Miller, S. M. (1989). Cognitive informational styles in the process of coping with threat and frustration. *Advances in Behaviour Research and Therapy, 11*, 223-234. doi:10.1016/0146-6402(89)90026-X

Miller, S. M. (1996). Monitoring and blunting of threatening information: Cognitive interference and facilitation in the coping process. In I. G. Sarason, G. R. Pierce, & B. R. Sarason (Eds.), *Cognitive interference: Theories, methods, and findings.* (pp. 175-190). Hillsdale, NJ: Lawrence Erlbaum Associates.

Miller, S. M., Fang, C. Y., Diefenbach, M. A., & Bales, C. B. (2001). Tailoring psychosocial interventions to the individual's health information-processing style: The influence of monitoring versus blunting in cancer risk and disease. In A. Baum & B. L. andersen (Eds.), *Psychosocial interventions for cancer.* (pp. 343-362). Washington, DC: American Psychological Association.

Miller, S. M., Fleisher, L., Roussi, P., Buzaglo, J., Schnoll, R., Slater, E., . . . Popa-Mabe, M. (2005). Facilitating informed decision making about breast cancer risk and genetic counseling among women calling the NCI's cancer information service. *Journal of Health Communication, 10*, 119-136. doi:10.1080/07366290500265335

Miller, W. R., & Rollnick, S. (2013). *Motivational interviewing: Helping people change (3rd ed.)*. New York: Guilford.

Mitchell, T., Dee, D. L., Phares, C. R., Lipman, H. B., Gould, L. H., Kutty, P., . . . Fishbein, D. B. (2011). Non-pharmaceutical interventions during an outbreak of 2009 pandemic influenza A (H1N1) virus infection at a large public university, April-May 2009. *Clinical Infectious Diseases, 52(Suppl 1)*, S138-S145.

Moraes, L. J., Miranda, M. B., Loures, L. F., Mainieri, A. G., & Mármora, C. H. C. (2017). A systematic review of psychoneuroimmunology-based interventions. *Psychology, Health & Medicine, 23*, 635-652.

Morens, D. M., & Fauci, A. S. (2017). Pandemic Zika: A formidable challenge to medicine and public health. *Journal of Infectious Diseases, 216*, S857-S859. doi:doi.org/10.1093/infdis/jix383

Morens, D. M., Taubenberger, J. K., & Fauci, A. S. (2008). Predominant role of bacterial pneumonia as a cause of death in pandemic influenza: Implications for pandemic influenza preparedness. *Journal of Infectious Diseases, 198*, 962-970. doi:10.1086/591708

Morens, D. M., Taubenberger, J. K., Folkers, G. K., & Fauci, A. S. (2010). Pandemic influenza's 500th anniversary. *Clinical Infectious Diseases, 51*, 1442-1444. doi:10.1086/657429

Moritz, S., & Pohl, R. F. (2009). Biased processing of threat-related information rather than knowledge deficits contributes to overestimation of threat in obsessive-compulsive disorder. *Behavior Modification, 33*, 763-777. doi:10.1177/0145445509344217

Morrell, H. E. R., Lapsley, D. K., & Halpern-Felsher, B. L. (2016). Subjective invulnerability and perceptions of tobacco-related benefits predict adolescent smoking behavior. *Journal of Early Adolescence, 36*, 679-703. doi:10.1177/0272431615578274

Moulding, R., Nix-Carnell, S., Schnabel, A., Nedeljkovic, M., Burnside, E. E., Lentini, A. F., ... Mehzabin, N. (2016). Better the devil you know than a world you don't? Intolerance of uncertainty and worldview explanations for belief in conspiracy theories. *Personality and Individual Differences, 98*, 345-354. doi:10.1016/j.paid.2016.04.060

Murray, D. R., & Schaller, M. (2012). Threat(s) and conformity deconstructed: Perceived threat of infectious disease and its implications for conformist attitudes and behavior. *European Journal of Social Psychology, 42*, 180-188. doi:10.1002/ejsp.863

Murray, D. R., & Schaller, M. (2016). The behavioral immune system: Implications for social cognition, social interaction, and social influence. *Advances in Experimental Social Psychology, 53*, 75-129. doi:10.1016/bs.aesp.2015.09.002

Muthusamy, N., Levine, T. R., & Weber, R. (2009). Scaring the already scared: Some problems with HIV/AIDS fear appeals in Namibia. *Journal of Communication, 59*, 317-344.

Muzzatti, S. L. (2005). Bits of falling sky and global pandemics: Moral panic and Severe Acute Respiratory Syndrome (SARS). *Illness, Crisis, & Loss, 13*, 117-128.

Nathan, P. E., & Gorman, J. M. (2015). *A guide to treatments that work (4th ed.)*. Oxford: Oxford University Press.

National Academy of Medicine. (2016). *The neglected dimension of global security: A framework to counter infectious disease crises*. Washington, DC: National Academies Press.

Navarrete, C. D., & Fessler, D. M. T. (2006). Disease avoidance and ethnocentrism: The effects of disease vulnerability and disgust sensitivity on intergroup attitudes. *Evolution and Human Behavior, 27*, 270-282.

Neria, Y., & Sullivan, G. M. (2011). Understanding the mental health effects of indirect exposure to mass trauma through the media. *Journal of the American Medical Association, 306*, 1374-1375. doi:10.1001/jama.2011.1358

Nerlich, B., & Halliday, C. (2007). Avian flu: The creation of expectations in the interplay between science and the media. *Sociology of Health & Illness, 29*, 46-65.

Newburn, T. (2016). Reflections on why riots don't happen. *Theoretical Criminology, 20*, 125-144. doi:10.1177/1362480615598829

Newport, F. (2015). In U.S., percentage saying vaccines are vital dips slightly. Retrieved 7 December, 2017, from http://www.gallup.com/poll/181844/percentage-saying-vaccines-vital-dips-slightly.aspx.

Nicas, M., & Jones, R. M. (2009). Relative contributions of four exposure pathways to influenza infection risk. *Risk Analysis, 29*, 1292-1303. doi:10.1111/j.1539-6924.2009.01253.x

Nishiura, H., & Inaba, H. (2011). Estimation of the incubation period of influenza A (H1N1-2009) among imported cases: Addressing censoring using outbreak data at the origin of importation. *Journal of Theoretical Biology, 272*, 123-130. doi:10.1016/j.jtbi.2010.12.017

Norkin, L. C. (2014). The 2004 flu vaccine shortage: Don't put all your eggs in one basket. https://norkinvirology.wordpress.com/2014/12/10/the-2004-flu-vaccine-shortage-dont-put-all-your-eggs-in-one-basket/, accessed January 29, 2019.

Norr, A. M., Albanese, B. J., Oglesby, M. E., Allan, N. P., & Schmidt, N. B. (2015). Anxiety sensitivity and intolerance of uncertainty as potential risk factors for cyberchondria. *Journal of Affective Disorders, 174*, 64-69. doi:10.1016/j.jad.2014.11.023

Norris, A. L., & Marcus, D. K. (2014). Cognition in health anxiety and hypochondriasis: Recent advances. *Current Psychiatry Reviews, 10*, 44-49. doi:10.2174/1573400509666131119004151

Norton, P. J., & Paulus, D. J. (2017). Transdiagnostic models of anxiety disorder: Theoretical and empirical underpinnings. *Clinical Psychology Review, 56*, 122-137. doi:10.1016/j.cpr.2017.03.004

O'Bryan, E. M., & McLeish, A. C. (2017). An examination of the indirect effect of intolerance of uncertainty on health anxiety through anxiety sensitivity physical concerns. *Journal of Psychopathology and Behavioral Assessment, 39*, 715-722. doi:10.1007/s10862-017-9613-y

O'Sullivan, T. L., & Phillips, K. P. (2019). From SARS to pandemic influenza: The framing of high-risk populations. *Natural Hazards*. doi:10.1007/s11069-019-03584-6

Oaten, M., Stevenson, R. J., & Case, T. I. (2009). Disgust as a disease avoidance mechanism. *Psychological Bulletin, 135*, 303-321.

Obsessive-Compulsive Cognitions Working Group. (2005). Psychometric validation of the obsessive belief questionnaire and interpretation of intrusions inventory—Part 2: Factor analyses and testing of a brief version. *Behaviour Research and Therapy, 43*, 1527-1542. doi:10.1016/j.brat.2004.07.010

Olatunji, B. O., Cisler, J., McKay, D., & Phillips, M. L. (2010). Is disgust associated with psychopathology? Emerging research in the anxiety disorders. *Psychiatry Research, 175*, 1-10. doi:10.1016/j.psychres.2009.04.007

Olatunji, B. O., & McKay, D. (2009). *Disgust and its disorders: Theory, assessment, and treatment implications*. Washington, DC: American Psychological Association.

Oliver, J. E., & Wood, T. (2014). Medical conspiracy theories and health behaviors in the United States. *JAMA Internal Medicine, 174*, 817-818. doi:10.1001/jamainternmed.2014.190

Oshitani, H. (2006). Potential benefits and limitations of various strategies to mitigate the impact of an influenza pandemic. *Journal of Infection and Chemotherapy, 12*, 167-171.

Öst, L.-G., & Sterner, U. (1987). Applied tension: A specific behavioral method for treatment of blood phobia. *Behaviour Research and Therapy, 25*, 25-29. doi:10.1016/0005-7967(87)90111-2

Pan-Canadian Public Health Network. (2016). *Canadian pandemic influenza preparedness*. Ottawa: Canadian Government Information Digital Preseveration Network.

Park, J. H., Faulkner, J., & Schaller, M. (2003). Evolved disease-avoidance processes and contemporary anti-social behavior: Prejudicial attitudes and avoidance of people with physical disabilities. *Journal of Nonverbal Behavior, 27*, 65-87. doi:10.1023/A:1023910408854

Park, J. H., Schaller, M., & Crandall, C. S. (2007). Pathogen-avoidance mechanisms and the stigmatization of obese people. *Evolution and Human Behavior, 28*, 410-414. doi:10.1016/j.evolhumbehav.2007.05.008

Parmet, W. E., & Sinha, M. S. (2017). A panic foretold: Ebola in the United States. *Critical Public Health, 27*, 148-155.

Parsons, S., Simmons, W., Shinhoster, F., & Kilburn, J. (1999). A test of the grapevine: An empirical examination of conspiracy theories among African Americans. *Sociological Spectrum, 19*, 201-222. doi:10.1080/027321799280235

Peters, G.-J. Y., Ruiter, R. A. C., & Kok, G. (2013). Threatening communication: A critical re-analysis and a revised meta-analytic test of fear appeal theory. *Health Psychology Review, 7 (Suppl. 1)*, S8-S31.

Petrie, K. J., Moss-Morris, R., Grey, C., & Shaw, M. (2004). The relationship of negative affect and perceived sensitivity to symptom reporting following vaccination. *British Journal of Health Psychology, 9*, 101-111. doi:10.1348/135910704322778759

Petrovska, B. B., & Cekovska, S. (2010). Extracts from the history and medical properties of garlic. *Pharmacognosy Review, 4*, 106-110. doi:10.4103/0973-7847.65321

Pettigrew, E. (1983). *The silent enemy: Canada and the deadly flu of 1918*. Saskatoon, SK: Western Producer Praire Books.

Pfattheicher, S., Strauch, C., Diefenbacher, S., & Schnuerch, R. (2018). A field study on watching eyes and hand hygiene compliance in a public restroom. *Journal of Applied Social Psychology, 48*, 188-194. doi:10.1111/jasp.12501

Phillips, A. C., Carroll, D., Burns, V. E., & Drayson, M. (2005). Neuroticism, cortisol reactivity, and antibody response to vaccination. *Psychophysiology, 42*, 232-238.

Pilkington, E., & Glenza, J. (2019). Facebook under pressure to halt rise of anti-vaccination groups. *The Guardian*, https://www.theguardian.com/technology/2019/feb/12/facebook-anti-vaxxer-vaccination-groups-pressure-misinformation?CMP=share_btn_link, accessed February 13, 2019.

Plans-Rubio, P. (2012). The vaccination coverage required to establish herd immunity against influenza viruses. *Preventive Medicine, 55*, 72-77.

Pless, A., McLennan, S. R., Nicca, D., Shaw, D. M., & Elger, B. S. (2017). Reasons why nurses decline influenza vaccination: A qualitative study. *BMC Nursing, 16*, article 20, DOI 10.1186/s12912-12017-10215-12915.

Prager, F., Wei, D., & Rose, A. (2017). Total economic consequences of an influenza outbreak in the United States. *Risk Analysis, 37*, 4-19. doi:10.1111/risa.12625

Pringle, H. (2015). How Europeans brought sickness to the New World. *Science*, online edition; http://www.sciencemag.org/news/2015/2006/how-europeans-brought-sickness-new-world.

Public Policy Polling. (2013). Democrats and Republicans differ on conspiracy theory beliefs. Retrieved March 3, 2018, https://www.publicpolicypolling.com/polls/democrats-and-republicans-differ-on-conspiracy-theory-beliefs/.

Quick, J. D. (2018). *The end of epidemics: The looming threat and how to stop it*. New York: St. Martin's Press.

Rains, S. A. (2013). The nature of psychological reactance revisited: A meta-analytic review. *Human Communication Research, 39*, 47-73. doi:10.1111/j.1468-2958.2012.01443.x

Ravert, R. D., Schwartz, S. J., Zamboanga, B. L., Kim, S. Y., Weisskirch, R. S., & Bersamin, M. (2009). Sensation seeking and danger invulnerability: Paths to college student risk-taking. *Personality and Individual Differences, 47*, 763-768. doi:10.1016/j.paid.2009.06.017

Remmerswaal, D., & Muris, P. (2011). Children's fear reactions to the 2009 Swine Flu pandemic: The role of threat information as provided by parents. *Journal of Anxiety Disorders, 25*, 444-449. doi:10.1016/j.janxdis.2010.11.008

Ricks, D. (2003). The flu factor in bioterrorism. *Newsday*, http://www.ph.ucla.edu/epi/bioter/flufactorbio.html, accessed February 4, 2019.

Riddell, R. P., Taddio, A., McMurtry, C. M., Chambers, C., Shah, V., & Noel, M. (2015). Psychological interventions for vaccine injections in young children 0 to 3 years: Systematic review of randomized controlled trials and quasi-randomized controlled trials. *Clinical Journal of Pain, 31*(10 Suppl), S64-S71. doi:10.1097/AJP.0000000000000279

Riddell, R. P., Taddio, A., McMurtry, C. M., Shah, V., Noel, M., & Chambers, C. T. (2015). Process interventions for vaccine injections: Systematic review of randomized controlled trials and quasi-randomized controlled trials. *Clinical Journal of Pain, 31*(10 Suppl), S99-S108. doi:10.1097/AJP.0000000000000280

Ritz, T., Meuret, A. E., & Alvord, M. K. (2014). Blood-injection-injury phobia. In L. Grossman & S. Walfish (Eds.), *Translating psychological research into practice* (pp. 295-301). New York: Springer.

Rosenberg, B. D., & Siegel, J. T. (2017). A 50-year review of psychological reactance theory: Do not read this article. *Motivation Science, 4*, 281-300. doi:10.1037/mot0000091

Rosnow, R. L., Esposito, J. L., & Gibney, L. (1988). Factors influencing rumor spreading: Replication and extension. *Language & Communication, 8*, 29-42. doi:10.1016/0271-5309(88)90004-3

Rosnow, R. L., & Fine, G. A. (1976). *Rumor and gossip: The social psychology of hearsay*. New York: Elsevier.

Rosser, B. A. (2018). Intolerance of uncertainty as a transdiagnostic mechanism of psychological difficulties: A systematic review of evidence pertaining to causality and temporal precedence. *Cognitive Therapy and Research*. doi:10.1007/s10608-018-9964-z

Rozin, P., Haidt, J., & McCauley, C. R. (2008). Disgust. In M. Lewis, J. M. Haviland-Jones, & L. F. Barrett (Eds.), *Handbook of emotions (3rd ed.)* (pp. 757-776). New York: Guilford.

Rubin, G. J., Amlôt, R., Page, L., & Wessely, S. (2009). Public perceptions, anxiety, and behaviour change in relation to the swine flu outbreak: Cross sectional telephone survey. *British Medical Journal, 339,* b2651. doi:10.1136/bmj.b2651

Rubin, G. J., & Wessely, S. (2013). The psychological and psychiatric effects of terrorism: Lessons from London. *Psychiatric Clinics of North America, 36,* 339-350.

Salkovskis, P. M., & Warwick, H. M. C. (2001). Meaning, misinterpretations, and medicine: A cognitive-behavioral approach to understanding health anxiety and hypochondriasis. In V. Starcevic, D. R. Lipsitt, V. Starcevic, & D. R. Lipsitt (Eds.), *Hypochondriasis: Modern perspectives on an ancient malady* (pp. 202-222). New York: Oxford University Press.

Sandman, P. M. (2009). Pandemics: Good hygiene is not enough. *Nature, 459,* 322-323.

Saxena, H. (2018). Are anxious patients causing the flu vax shortage by having two shots? *Pharmacy News,* https://www.pharmacynews.com.au/news/are-anxious-patients-causing-flu-vax-shortage-having-two-shots, accessed January 29, 2019.

Schaller, M., & Park, J. H. (2011). The behavioral immune system (and why it matters). *Current Directions in Psychological Science, 20,* 99-103.

Schibalski, J. V., Müller, M., Ajdacic-Gross, V., Vetter, S., Rodgers, S., Oexle, N., . . . Rüsch, N. (2017). Stigma-related stress, shame and avoidant coping reactions among members of the general population with elevated symptom levels. *Comprehensive Psychiatry, 74,* 224-230. doi:10.1016/j.comppsych.2017.02.001

Schmidt, N. B., Lerew, D. R., & Trakowski, J. H. (1997). Body vigilance in panic disorder: Evaluating attention to bodily perturbations. *Journal of Consulting and Clinical Psychology, 65,* 214-220. doi:10.1037/0022-006X.65.2.214

Schoch-Spana, M. (2004). Lessons from the 1918 pandemic influenza: Psychosocial consequences of a catastrophic outbreak of disease. In R. J. Ursano, A. E. Norwood, & C. S. Fullerton (Eds.), *Bioterrorism: Psychological and public health interventions* (pp. 38-55). New York: Cambridge University Press.

Setbon, M., & Raude, J. (2010). Factors in vaccination intention against the pandemic influenza A/H1N1. *European Journal of Public Health, 20,* 490-494.

Sharma, M., Yadav, K., Yadav, N., & Ferdinand, K. C. (2017). Zika virus pandemic-analysis of Facebook as a social media health information platform. *American Journal of Infection Control, 45*, 301-302. doi:10.1016/j.ajic.2016.08.022

Sharot, T., Korn, C. W., & Dolan, R. J. (2011). How unrealistic optimism is maintained in the face of reality. *Nature Neuroscience, 14*, 1475-1479. doi:10.1038/nn.2949

Shattuck, E. C., & Muehlenbein, M. P. (2016). Towards an integrative picture of human sickness behavior. *Brain, Behavior, and Immunity, 57*, 255-262. doi:10.1016/j.bbi.2016.05.002

Shear, M. K., & Gribbin Bloom, C. (2017). Complicated grief treatment: An evidence-based approach to grief therapy. *Journal of Rational-Emotive & Cognitive-Behavior Therapy, 35*, 6-25. doi:10.1007/s10942-016-0242-2

Shen, Z., Ning, F., Zhou, W., He, X., Lin, C., Chin, D. P., . . . Schuchat, A. (2004). Superspreading SARS events, Beijing, 2003. *Emerging Infectious Diseases, 10*, 256-260.

Shepperd, J. A., Waters, E. A., Weinstein, N. D., & Klein, W. M. P. (2015). A primer on unrealistic optimism. *Current Directions in Psychological Science, 24*, 232-237. doi:10.1177/0963721414568341

Shibutani, T. (1966). *Improvised news: A sociological study of rumor*. New York: Bobbs-Merrill.

Shihata, S., McEvoy, P. M., Mullan, B. A., & Carleton, R. N. (2016). Intolerance of uncertainty in emotional disorders: What uncertainties remain? *Journal of Anxiety Disorders, 41*, 115-124. doi:10.1016/j.janxdis.2016.05.001

Shultz, J. M., Baingana, F., & Neria, Y. (2015). The 2014 Ebola outbreak and mental health: Current status and recommended response. *Journal of the American Medical Association, 313*, 567-568. doi:10.1001/jama.2014.17934

Shultz, J. M., Espinel, Z., Flynn, B. W., Hoffmann, Y., & Cohen, R. E. (2008). *DEEP PREP: All-hazards disaster behavioral health training*. Miami, FL: DEEP Center.

Simpson, A. W. (1985). Quackery and contract law: The case of the carbolic smoke ball. *Journal of Legal Studies, 14*, 345-389.

Skene, K. J., Paltiel, A. D., Shim, E., & Galvani, A. P. (2014). A marginal benefit approach for vaccinating influenza "superspreaders". *Medical Decision Making, 34*, 536-549. doi:10.1177/0272989X14523502

Slovic, P., Finucane, M. L., Peters, E., & MacGregor, D. G. (2004). Risk as analysis and risk as feelings: Some thoughts about affect, reason, risk, and rationality. *Risk Analysis, 24*, 311-322. doi:10.1111/j.0272-4332.2004.00433.x

Slovic, P., Finucane, M. L., Peters, E., & MacGregor, D. G. (2007). The affect heuristic. *European Journal of Operational Research, 177*, 1333-1352.

Smallman, S. (2015). Whom do you trust? Doubt and conspiracy theories in the 2009 influenza pandemic. *Journal of International & Global Studies, 6*, 1-24.

Smith, B. W., Kay, V. S., Hoyt, T. V., & Bernard, M. L. (2009). Predicting the anticipated emotional and behavioral responses to an avian flu outbreak. *American Journal of Infection Control, 37*, 371-380. doi:10.1016/j.ajic.2008.08.007

Soper, G. A. (1939). The curious career of Typhoid Mary. *Bulletin of the New York Academy of Medicine, 15*, 698-712.

Sørensen, K., Van den Broucke, S., Fullam, J., Doyle, G., Pelikan, J., Slonska, Z., & Brand, H. (2012). Health literacy and public health: A systematic review and integration of definitions and models. *BMC Public Health, 12*, 80-80. doi:10.1186/1471-2458-12-80

Spielberger, C. D. (1979). *Understanding stress and anxiety*. New York: Harper & Row.

Spoont, M. R., Williams, J. W., Jr., Kehle-Forbes, S., Nieuwsma, J. A., Mann-Wrobel, M. C., & Gross, R. (2015). Does this patient have posttraumatic stress disorder? Rational clinical examination systematic review. *Journal of the American Medical Association, 314*, 501-510. doi:10.1001/jama.2015.7877

Staiano, J. (2008). The impact of plague on human behavior in seventeeth century Europe. *ESSAI, 6*, article 6, http://dc.cod.edu/essai/vol6/iss1/46.

Statistics Canada. (2010). *Community Health Survey*. Retrieved July 19, 2018 from http://www.statcan.gc.ca/daily-quotidien/100719/dq100719beng.htm.

Stead, M., Critchlow, N., Eadie, D., Sullivan, F., Gravenhorst, K., & Dobbie, F. (2019). Mandatory policies for influenza vaccination: Views of managers and healthcare workers in England. *Vaccine, 37*, 69-75. doi:10.1016/j.vaccine.2018.11.033

Stebbins, S., Downs, J. S., & Vukotich, C. J., Jr. (2009). Using nonpharmaceutical interventions to prevent influenza transmission in elementary school children: Parent and teacher perspectives. *Journal of Public Health Management and Practice, 15*, 112-117.

SteelFisher, G. K., Blendon, R. J., Ward, J. R. M., Rapoport, R., Kahn, E. B., & Kohl, K. S. (2012). Public response to the 2009 influenza A H1N1 pandemic: A polling study in five countries. *Lancet Infectious Diseases, 12*, 845-850.

Stoeber, J. (2018). *The psychology of perfectionism: Theory, research, applications.* New York: Taylor & Francis.

Strekalova, Y. A. (2017). Health risk information engagement and amplification on social media: News about an emerging pandemic on Facebook. *Health Education & Behavior, 44*, 332-339. doi:10.1177/1090198116660310

Sunderland, M., Newby, J. M., & Andrews, G. (2013). Health anxiety in Australia: Prevalence, comorbidity, disability and service use. *British Journal of Psychiatry, 202*, 56-61. doi:10.1192/bjp.bp.111.103960

Swami, V., Voracek, M., Stieger, S., Tran, U. S., & Furnham, A. (2014). Analytic thinking reduces belief in conspiracy theories. *Cognition, 133*, 572-585. doi:10.1016/j.cognition.2014.08.006

Swift, A. (2013). Majority in U.S. still believe JFK killed in a conspiracy, https://news.gallup.com/poll/165893/majority-believe-jfk-killed-conspiracy.aspx, accessed April 2, 2019.

Taddio, A., Ipp, M., Thivakaran, S., Jamal, A., Parikh, C., Smart, S., . . . Katz, J. (2012). Survey of the prevalence of immunization non-compliance due to needle fears in children and adults. *Vaccine, 30*, 4807-4812. doi:10.1016/j.vaccine.2012.05.011

Taha, S., Matheson, K., & Anisman, H. (2013). The 2009 H1N1 influenza pandemic: The role of threat, coping, and media trust on vaccination intentions in Canada. *Journal of Health Communication, 18*, 278-290. doi:10.1080/10810730.2012.727960

Taha, S., Matheson, K., Cronin, T., & Anisman, H. (2014). Intolerance of uncertainty, appraisals, coping, and anxiety: The case of the 2009 H1N1 pandemic. *British Journal of Health Psychology, 19*, 592-605. doi:10.1111/bjhp.12058

Tang, L., Bie, B., Park, S.-E., & Zhi, D. (2018). Social media and outbreaks of emerging infectious diseases: A systematic review of literature. *American Journal of Infection Control, 46*, 962-972. doi:10.1016/j.ajic.2018.02.010

Taubenberger, J. K., & Morens, D. M. (2006). 1918 influenza: The mother of all pandemics. *Emerging Infectious Diseases, 12*, 15-22.

Taubenberger, J. K., Reid, A. H., Janczewski, T. A., & Fanning, T. G. (2001). Integrating historical, clinical and molecular genetic data in order to explain the origin and virulence of the 1918 Spanish influenza virus.

Philosophical Transactions of The Royal Society of London. Series B, Biological Sciences, 356, 1829-1839.

Taylor, S. (2017). *Clinician's guide to PTSD (2nd ed.).* New York: Guildford.

Taylor, S. (2019). Anxiety sensitivity. In J. S. Abramowitz & S. M. Blakey (Eds.), *Clinical handbook of fear and anxiety: Psychological processes and treatment mechanisms.* Washington, DC: American Psychological Association.

Taylor, S., & Asmundson, G. J. G. (2004). *Treating health anxiety.* New York: Guilford.

Taylor, S., & Asmundson, G. J. G. (2017). Treatment of health anxiety. In E. Storch, J. S. Abramowitz, & D. McKay (Eds.), *Handbook of obsessive-compulsive disorders: Vol. 2: Obsessive-compulsive related disorders* (pp. 977-989). Chichester: Wiley.

Taylor, S., Asmundson, G. J. G., & Coons, M. J. (2005). Current directions in the treatment of hypochondriasis. *Journal of Cognitive Psychotherapy, 19,* 285-304. doi:10.1891/jcop.2005.19.3.285

Taylor, S., Zvolensky, M. J., Cox, B. J., Deacon, B., Heimberg, R. G., Ledley, D. R., . . . Cardenas, S. J. (2007). Robust dimensions of anxiety sensitivity: Development and initial validation of the Anxiety Sensitivity Index-3. *Psychological Assessment, 19,* 176-188. doi:10.1037/1040-3590.19.2.176

Taylor, S. E., & Brown, J. D. (1988). Illusion and well-being: A social psychological perspective on mental health. *Psychological Bulletin, 103,* 193-210. doi:10.1037/0033- 2909.103.2.193

Temime, L., Opatowski, L., Pannet, Y., Brun-Buisson, C., Boëlle, P. Y., & Guillemot, D. (2009). Peripatetic health-care workers as potential superspreaders. *Proceedings of the National Academy of Sciences, 106,* 18420-18425. doi:10.1073/pnas.0900974106

Thibodeau, M. A., Carleton, R. N., McEvoy, P. M., Zvolensky, M. J., Brandt, C. P., Boelen, P. A., . . . Asmundson, G. J. G. (2015). Developing scales measuring disorder-specific intolerance of uncertainty (DSIU): A new perspective on transdiagnostic. *Journal of Anxiety Disorders, 31,* 49-57. doi:10.1016/j.janxdis.2015.01.006

Thomas, Y., Vogel, G., Wunderli, W., Suter, P., Witschi, M., Koch, D., . . . Kaiser, L. (2008). Survival of influenza virus on banknotes. *Applied and Environmental Microbiology, 74,* 3002-3007.

Trepte, S., & Scharkow, M. (2017). Friends and lifesavers: How social capital and social support received in media environments contribute to well-being. In L. Reinecke & M. B. Oliver (Eds.), *The Routledge handbook of media use and well-being: International perspectives on theory and research on positive media effects.* (pp. 304-316). New York: Routledge.

Trope, Y., & Liberman, N. (2010). Construal level theory of psychological distance. *Psychological Review, 117,* 440-463.

Tufekci, Z., & Freelon, D. (2013). Introduction to the special issue on new media and social unrest. *American Behavioral Scientist, 57,* 843-847. doi:10.1177/0002764213479376

Tuite, A. R., Greer, A. L., Whelan, M., Winter, A.-L., Lee, B., Yan, P., . . . Fisman, D. N. (2010). Estimated epidemiologic parameters and morbidity associated with pandemic H1N1 influenza. *Canadian Medical Association Journal, 182,* 131-136. doi:10.1503/cmaj.091807

Tversky, A., & Kahneman, D. (1973). Availability: A heuristic for judging frequency and probability. *Cognitive Psychology, 5,* 207-232.

Tyrer, P., & Tyrer, H. (2018). Health anxiety: Detection and treatment. *British Journal of Psychiatry Advances, 24,* 66-72. doi:10.1192/bja.2017.5

U.S. Congress Joint Economic Committee. (2010). *Expanding access to paid sick leave: The impact of the healthy families act on America's workers.* Washington, DC: Author.

van den Bulck, J., & Custers, K. (2009). Television exposure is related to fear of avian flu, an ecological study across 23 member states of the European Union. *European Journal of Public Health, 19,* 370-374. doi:10.1093/eurpub/ckp061

van Dijk, S. D. M., Hanssen, D., Naarding, P., Lucassen, P., Comijs, H., & Oude Voshaar, R. (2016). Big Five personality traits and medically unexplained symptoms in later life. *European Psychiatry, 38,* 23-30. doi:10.1016/j.eurpsy.2016.05.002

van Prooijen, J.-W., & van Vugt, M. (2018). Conspiracy theories: Evolved functions and psychological mechanisms. *Perspectives on Psychological Science, 13,* 770-788. doi:10.1177/1745691618774270

Vandenbos, G. R. (Ed.) (2007). *APA dictionary of psychology.* Washington, DC: American Psychological Association.

Vander Haegen, M., & Etienne, A.-M. (2016). Cognitive processes across anxiety disorders related to intolerance of uncertainty: Clinical review. *Cogent Psychology, 3,* doi:10.1080/23311908.23312016.21215773.

Vietri, J. T., Meng, L., Galvani, A. P., & Chapman, G. B. (2011). Vaccinating to help ourselves and others. *Medical Decision Making, 12,* 447-458.

Virlogeux, V., Yang, J., Fang, V. J., Feng, L., Tsang, T. K., Jiang, H., . . . Cowling, B. J. (2016). Association between the severity of influenza A(H7N9) virus infections and length of the incubation period. *PLoS ONE, 11*, e0148506. doi:10.1371/journal.pone.0148506

Wain, J., Hendriksen, R. S., Mikoleit, M. L., Keddy, K. H., & Ochiai, R. L. (2015). Typhoid fever. *Lancet, 385*, 1136-1145. doi:10.1016/S0140-6736(13)62708-7

Wainberg, M. A. (2008). HIV transmission should be decriminalized: HIV prevention programs depend on it. *Retrovirology, 5*, 108-108. doi:10.1186/1742-4690-5-108

Wald, P. (2008). *Contagious: Cultures, carriers, and the outbreak narrative*. Durham, NC: Duke University Press.

Walker, J. (2016). Civil society's role in a public health crisis. *Issues in Science & Technology, 32*, 43-48.

Wang, T. L., Jing, L., & Bocchini, J. A., Jr. (2017). Mandatory influenza vaccination for all healthcare personnel: A review on justification, implementation and effectiveness. *Current Opinion in Pediatrics, 29*, 606-615. doi:10.1097/MOP.0000000000000527

Washer, P. (2004). Representations of SARS in the British newspapers. *Social Science and Medicine, 59*, 2561-2571. doi:10.1016/j.socscimed.2004.03.038

Watson, D., & O'Hara, M. W. (2017). *Understanding the emotional disorders*. New York: Oxford University Press.

Watt, H. (2017). Man found guilty of trying to infect 10 Grindr dates with HIV. *The Guardian,* https://www.theguardian.com/uk-news/2017/nov/15/hairdresser-found-guilty-of-trying-to-infect-10-men-he-met-on-grindr-with-hiv, accessed February 4, 2019.

Webby, R. J., & Webster, R. G. (2003). Are we ready for pandemic influenza? *Science, 302*, 1519-1522.

Webster, R. G., & Govorkova, E. A. (2006). H5N1 Influenza—Continuing evolution and spread. *New England Journal of Medicine, 355*, 2174-2177.

Weigmann, K. (2018). The genesis of a conspiracy theory: Why do people believe in scientific conspiracy theories and how do they spread? *EMBO Reports, 19*, doi:10.15252/embr.201845935

Weinstein, N. (1980). Unrealistic optimism about future life events. *Journal of Personality and Social Psychology, 39*, 806-820.

Wheaton, M. G., Abramowitz, J. S., Berman, N. C., Fabricant, L. E., & Olatunji, B. O. (2012). Psychological predictors of anxiety in response to the H1N1 (swine flu) pandemic. *Cognitive Therapy and Research, 36*, 210-218. doi:10.1007/s10608-011-9353-3

Wheaton, M. G., Berman, N. C., Franklin, J. C., & Abramowitz, J. S. (2010). Health anxiety: Latent structure and associations with anxiety-related psychological processes. *Journal of Psychopathology and Behavioral Assessment, 32,* 565-574. doi:10.1007/s10862-010-9179-4

White, A. E., Johnson, K. A., & Kwan, V. S. Y. (2014). Four ways to infect me: Spatial, temporal, social, and probability distance influence evaluations of disease threat. *Social Cognition, 32,* 239-255. doi:10.1521/soco.2014.32.3.239

Wildoner, D. A. (2016). What's new with pandemic flu. *Clinical Microbiology Newsletter, 38,* 27-31. doi:10.1016/j.clinmicnews.2016.02.001

Williams, L., Rasmussen, S., Kleczkowski, A., Maharaj, S., & Cairns, N. (2015). Protection motivation theory and social distancing behaviour in response to a simulated infectious disease epidemic. *Psychology, Health & Medicine, 20,* 832-837.

Wilson, J. M., Iannarone, M., & Wang, C. (2009). Media reporting of the emergence of the 1968 influenza pandemic in Hong Kong: Implications for modern-day situational awareness. *Disaster Medicine & Public Health Preparedness, 3*(Suppl 2), S148-S153. doi:10.1097/DMP.0b013e3181abd603

Witte, K. (1992). Putting the fear back into fear appeals: Reconciling the literature. *Communication Monographs, 59,* 329-349.

Witte, K., & Allen, M. (2000). A meta-analysis of fear appeals: Implications for effective public health campaigns. *Health Education & Behavior, 27,* 591-615.

Witthöft, M., Kerstner, T., Ofer, J., Mier, D., Rist, F., Diener, C., & Bailer, J. (2016). Cognitive biases in pathological health anxiety: The contribution of attention, memory, and evaluation processes. *Clinical Psychological Science, 4,* 464-479. doi:10.1177/2167702615593474

Wiwanitkit, V. (2015). New atypical influenza: Possible trend for bioterrorism. *Journal of Bioterrorism and Biodefense, 6,* e119. doi: 110.4172/2157-2526.1000e4119.

Wong, L. P., & Sam, I. C. (2011). Knowledge and attitudes in regard to pandemic influenza A(H1N1) in a multiethnic community of Malaysia. *International Journal of Behavioral Medicine, 18,* 112-121.

Wood, M. J. (2018). Propagating and debunking conspiracy theories on Twitter during the 2015–2016 Zika virus outbreak. *Cyberpsychology, Behavior, and Social Networking, 21,* 485-490. doi:10.1089/cyber.2017.0669

Woolhouse, M. E., Dye, C., Etard, J. F., Smith, T., Charlwood, J. D., Garnett, G. P., . . . Anderson, R. M. (1997). Heterogeneities in the transmission of infectious agents: Implications for the design of control programs. *Proceedings of the National Academy of Sciences, 94*, 338-342.

World Health Organization. (2004). Summary of probable SARS cases with onset of illness from 1 November 2002 to 31 July 2003, http://www.who.int/csr/sars/country/table2004_04_21/en/, accessed July 27, 2018.

World Health Organization. (2005). *WHO checklist for influenza pandemic preparedness planning*. Geneva: Author.

World Health Organization. (2008). *WHO outbreak communication planning guide*. Geneva: Author.

World Health Organization. (2010a). Pandemic (H1N1) 2009. Frequently asked questions: What can I do? Retrieved from http://www.who.int/csr/disease/swineflu/frequently_asked_questions/what/en/

World Health Organization. (2010b). What is a pandemic? http://www.who.int/csr/disease/swineflu/frequently_asked_questions/pandemic/en/, accessed September 14, 2017.

World Health Organization. (2012). Vaccines against influenza WHO position paper. *Weekly Epidemiological Record, 87*, 461-476.

World Health Organization. (2019). Ten threats to global health in 2019. https://www.who.int/emergencies/ten-threats-to-global-health-in-2019, accessed February 25, 2019.

World Health Organization Writing Group. (2006). Nonpharmaceutical interventions for pandemic influenza, national and community measures. *Emerging Infectious Diseases, 12*, 88-94.

Wu, B. P., & Chang, L. (2012). The social impact of pathogen threat: How disease salience influences conformity. *Personality and Individual Differences, 53*, 50-54.

Wu, J. T., Cowling, B. J., Lau, E. H. Y., Ip, D. K. M., Ho, L.-M., Tsang, T., . . . Riley, S. (2010). School closure and mitigation of pandemic (H1N1) 2009, Hong Kong. *Emerging Infectious Diseases, 16*, 538-541. doi:10.3201/eid1603.091216

Wu, K. K., Chan, S. K., & Ma, T. M. (2005). Posttraumatic stress, anxiety, and depression in survivors of severe acute respiratory syndrome (SARS). *Journal of Traumatic Stress, 18*, 39-42.

Wu, P., Fang, Y., Guan, Z., Fan, B., Kong, J., Yao, Z., . . . Hoven, C. W. (2009). The psychological impact of the SARS epidemic on hospital employees in China. *Canadian Journal of Psychiatry, 54*, 302-311.

Xie, X.-F., Stone, E., Zheng, R., & Zhang, R.-G. (2011). The "Typhoon Eye Effect": Determinants of distress during the SARS epidemic. *Journal of Risk Research, 14*, 1091-1107.

Yaqub, O., Castle-Clarke, S., Sevdalis, N., & Chataway, J. (2014). Attitudes to vaccination: A critical review. *Social Science & Medicine, 112*, 1-11. doi:10.1016/j.socscimed.2014.04.018

Young, M. E., Norman, G. R., & Humphreys, K. R. (2008). Medicine in the popular press: The influence of the media on perceptions of disease. *PLoS ONE, 3*, e3552. doi:10.1371/journal.pone.0003552

Yun, G. W., Morin, D., Park, S., Joa, C. Y., Labbe, B., Lim, J., . . . Hyun, D. (2016). Social media and flu: Media Twitter accounts as agenda setters. *International Journal of Medical Informatics, 91*, 67-73. doi:10.1016/j.ijmedinf.2016.04.009

Zhu, X., Levasseur, P. R., Michaelis, K. A., Burfeind, K. G., & Marks, D. L. (2016). A distinct brain pathway links viral RNA exposure to sickness behavior. *Scientific Reports, 6*, 29885-29885. doi:10.1038/srep29885

Zipprich, J., Winter, K., Hacker, J., Xia, D., Watt, J., & Harriman, K. (2015). Measles outbreak—California, December 2014-February 2015. *Morbidity and Mortality Weekly Report, 64*, 373-376.

INDEX